A Daily Difference

How Ordinary People Can Do Extraordinary Things!

OR

How to integrate charitable giving into your daily life by doing small things each day to help those who are less fortunate and really need your help

Bob Zachmeier

Out of the Box Books
Tucson, Arizona

This publication contains the opinions, ideas, and personal experiences of its author. It is sold with the understanding that neither the author nor the publisher is engaged in rendering legal, tax, investment, insurance, financial, accounting, or other professional advice or services. If the reader requires such advice or services, a competent professional should be consulted. Relevant laws vary from state to state. The strategies outlined in this book may not be suitable for every individual, and are not guaranteed or warranted to produce any particular results. No warranty is made with respect to the accuracy or completeness of the information contained herein, and both the author and the publisher specifically disclaim any responsibility for any liability, loss, or risk, personal or otherwise, which is incurred as a consequence, directly or indirectly, of the use and application of any of the contents of this book.

Copyright © 2012 by Bob Zachmeier

All rights reserved, including the right of reproduction in whole or in part in any form.

ISBN: 978-0-9801855-4-6

Library of Congress Control Number:
2012903096

For information on other books by Bob Zachmeier
visit the publisher's website at:
www.outoftheboxbooks.com

When it comes to books… think Out of the Box!

Out of the Box Books
P.O. Box 64878, Tucson, AZ 85728

For Bill and BettyJo Zachmeier

I was blessed to have parents who expected great things from me. I now expect the same things from myself. Together, they gave me the confidence to set aggressive goals, the discipline to achieve them, and the desire to share my blessings with others.

"Charity begins at home, but should not end there."
- Thomas Fuller

Table of Contents

ACKNOWLEDGEMENTS	ix
INTRODUCTION	xi
CHAPTER 1 – Believing in Abundance	1
CHAPTER 2 – Fun with Flamingos	9
CHAPTER 3 – Cookies For Campers	19
CHAPTER 4 – A Blue Öyster Birthday	27
CHAPTER 5 – Caring Kids	35
CHAPTER 6 – Power in Numbers	43
CHAPTER 7 – Change From Lunch	51
CHAPTER 8 – Everyone Can Do Something	61
CHAPTER 9 – Follow the Leader	67
CHAPTER 10 – Creative Fundraising	75
CHAPTER 11 – Leaving Footprints	81
CHAPTER 12 – Dream Maker	87

TABLE OF CONTENTS

CHAPTER 13 – Creating Hope   93

CHAPTER 14 – The Gift of Compassion   103

CHAPTER 15 – A Dollar A Day   109

CHAPTER 16 – Small Change, Big Difference   115

CHAPTER 17 – Passionate Planning   121

CHAPTER 18 – Get Optimistic!   127

CHAPTER 19 – Challenge Yourself!   133

INDEX   139

About the Author   143

TABLE OF CONTENTS

Figures in This Book

1-1	Real Estate Sales 2000 - 2010	3
1-2	How Events Affect Our Actions	7
2-1	You've Been FLOCKED! Notice	11
2-2	Anti-Flocking Insurance Certificate	12
2-3	Soldier's Pocket Card	16
2-4	Miley Pickell	17
4-1	Blue Öyster Cult Poster	29
4-2	Blue Öyster Cult Backstage	30
4-3	Blue Öyster Cult Concert Photo	32
5-1	Lizzie Bell and Bob Zachmeier	37
5-2	Camden Garcia	41
6-1	REO4Kids Marketing Flyer	45
6-2	REO4Kids Exhibitor Booth	46
6-3	REO Insider Article	47
7-1	Conference Room Banner	55
7-2	Client Donation Flyer	57

TABLE OF CONTENTS

9-1	Ryan Hill Team in Mississippi	70
9-2	Teresa Ryan with Second Grade Class	72
10-1	Kelly and Samantha	80
13-1	Alex Blackwood	96
14-1	Lauren Border and Ebony	107

ACKNOWLEDGEMENTS

This book was easy to write because every person in it is a friend whose story I know from living through it with them. I did the majority of the writing for this book while on vacation for a week in Cabo San Lucas, Mexico, with my wife, Camille, my Mom, Betty Jo Zachmeier, and her husband, Roger Peet.

I thank God for blessing me with the ability to attract great people. Through many challenges, I have always prevailed due to the love and support of my friends and family. I am surrounded by the best group of people on earth!

I thank my wife, Camille, who patiently sat by me on vacation, reading as I wrote, and awakened as I came to bed after many late-night editing sessions well after midnight.

I thank my parents. Dad taught me to see things as they *could be* rather than as they are. His *vision* and my Mom's optimism are alive and well in me today. Although Dad passed away in 1996, Mom is still actively experiencing life.

I thank my brother, Mike, for bringing a unique and valuable perspective to our business and for helping to edit all of my books. He was always a straight A student who made me look bad, but now his perfectionism is coming in handy!

I thank Bryan Pellican for readily sharing his knowledge to help us achieve sales levels we never imagined possible.

I thank my friends in REO4Kids who took time to share their stories in this book, Amy Coleman and Bruce Hammer in Sacramento, CA, Lester Cox in Tempe, AZ, Teresa Ryan in Naperville, IL, Nancy Braun in Charlotte, NC, Pat Koch in San Diego, CA, Terry Rasner-Yacenda in Reno, NV, and Steven and Cindi Blackwood in Little Rock, AR. This giving group of people continues to inspire me on a daily basis.

ACKNOWLEDGEMENTS

I thank Ramsey Fahel for 20 years of friendship, encouragement, and thought-provoking conversation.

I thank Ron Gamble, Todd & Kathy Dirkschneider, and Harold & Hazel Copenhaver for their work at Montlure.

I thank Tom and Naomi Moon for REObroker.com, a network of caring people with a *Pay it Forward* attitude. Their support of our fundraising endeavors is truly appreciated.

I thank Joann Bersell, Debbie Turner, Kim Moss, Julie Benson, Catherine Alameda, Lauren Duffy, and Tori Bentley for their support of our silent auction and real estate closings.

I thank Eric Bloom for his work with Make-A-Wish® and the rest of Blue Öyster Cult for the discounted performance.

I thank Lizzie Bell, Camden Garcia, and their parents, Mike & Kathy Bell and Gil & Carol Garcia. These awesome families have worked through serious health issues by constantly looking to help others. They are an inspiration!

I thank John Fox in Tucson, AZ, Gena Foster in Jackson, MI, and Lauren Border in Dallas, TX, for their passionate desire to make the world a better place, one person at a time!

I thank Ken Blevins at PMH Financial for creating a company culture of sharing, matching employee gifts to local charities, and allowing employees to choose who they support.

I thank the generations of people who've given freely of their time, talents, and financial resources to benefit others. Their gifts of love and their compassion for their fellow human beings have set an example for the rest of us to follow.

I thank Amanda Smiklas and Joel Trupiano for getting us involved in the Optimist Club and I'd like to thank the people who read this book, become inspired by the people in it, and take action to help those around them. Sharing your blessings with others is the greatest blessing of all!

INTRODUCTION

People sometimes ask me why I share with others. I guess I hadn't thought about it much; it's just something my parents always did and that I want to do. My wife, Camille, feels the same way. My mother was in charge of our family's finances and before any of my five siblings or I received our allowance, we had to sit down with Mom to calculate how much we had earned. She wanted us to equate work with money so we would understand that effort is required to obtain a financial reward.

Each week Mom would review the chores that each of us completed, clarify the amount that each task paid, and then calculate how much allowance had been earned. It was always very clear that if you wanted more money you simply did more work. Our allowance was never an entitlement.

After determining how much was owed, Mom would open her purse and count out the exact amount. The money was then divided into three different piles that contained 10%, 50%, and 40%, respectively; the process was always the same.

First we'd gather up the money in the 10% pile and place it into a church donation envelope. All six of us had our own box of church envelopes and I can clearly remember watching each of my siblings make their own contribution as the collection basket was passed every Sunday.

Next, we'd take the 50% pile and place it into an envelope to be deposited at the bank during the next trip to

INTRODUCTION

town. Mom had opened a savings account for each of us when we were eight years old so we could start saving for college.

The remaining 40% was placed in our coin purse which was kept in an upper kitchen cabinet out of sight. We each had a handwritten piece of paper inside our coin purse with our money. Although we were allowed to make our own decisions about how we spent the money, we were responsible for documenting the expenditure so Mom could review what we'd purchased the next time our allowance was paid. The 50% I saved for college from my meager allowance and after-school jobs was enough to pay cash for my entire first year of tuition, room, and board.

Consistent contributions over time can produce a huge amount of money. My Dad earned less than $3,000 per year when he first started his job at the oil refinery in my hometown of Mandan, North Dakota. He and Mom religiously (no pun intended) gave 10% to the church and saved 10% of their gross pay for retirement while raising six children. They never made an exception in thirty-five years other than to increase the amount they saved and donated. Their will-power has always been an inspiration to me!

Initially, my parents' rate of savings was less than $1 per day, but each time Dad received a pay increase, they increased their savings accordingly. Over thirty-five years they amassed over $1 million dollars, while giving as much to the church as they saved! You can do the same thing through consistent saving, discipline, and the willingness to make a difference.

1

Believing in Abundance

"God has given us two hands, one to receive with and the other to give with. – Billy Graham"

A DAILY DIFFERENCE

More than twenty years ago I was walking through a shopping mall in Dallas, Texas, with my friend, Ramsey Fahel. As we walked and visited, Ramsey reached into his pocket and pulled out a handful of loose change. Every few steps he would drop one or two coins and continued to do so until all of the coins were gone.

I watched as the coins rolled under benches, against planters, and in ever-slowing circles on the spacious polished floors of the mall. Some people walked past without noticing while others scurried around picking up the coins that had settled near them. When the commotion had diminished, I turned to Ramsey and asked him why he had done that. Without thinking he replied, "To make someone's day better."

I started thinking of all the directions the coins had taken and began wondering how long it would take a cleaning attendant or child to find some of the coins that had rolled into obscure places. Ramsey must have dropped more than fifty coins, so I think that his gift made a LOT of people's day better and would continue to do so as more coins were found.

This story is the epitome of what charitable giving is about. All it takes is one person who cares enough to help. The good deeds of one person inspire others to do something kind, which inspires even more people until soon an epidemic breaks out!

Many people who give to others choose to give anonymously. It's quite noble to help someone without expecting a reward or even a "thank you" but when this is

CHAPTER 1 – BELIEVING IN ABUNDANCE

done, only the person receiving the gift is inspired. The compounding opportunity to inspire others, who inspire others, who inspire others, is forever lost. One simple act can inspire hundreds or even thousands of people to make a difference for those around them but if it's kept a secret, it dies.

I've convinced several of the most generous people I know to share their stories in this book. Learning how other ordinary people have found a way to fit charitable giving into their everyday lives will hopefully inspire you to either imitate their example or find your own way to help others.

Figure 1-1 Real Estate Sales 2000 – 2010

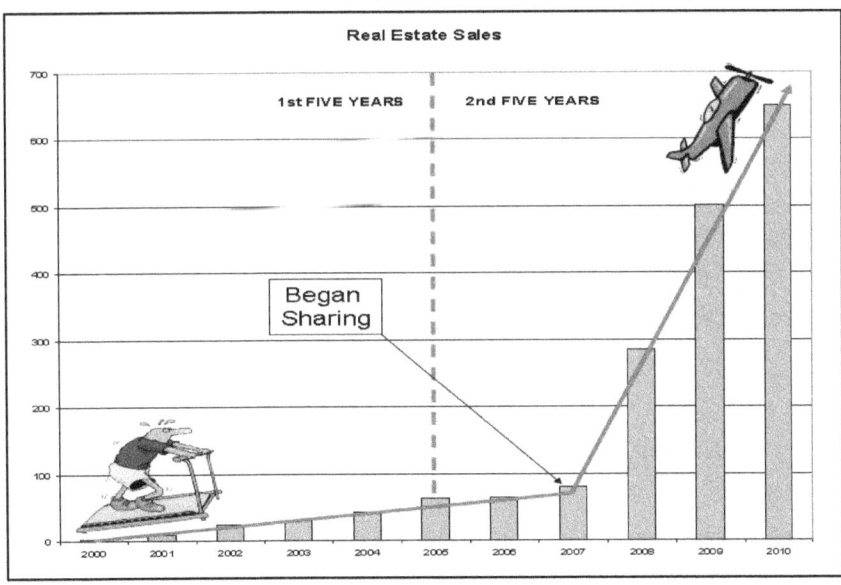

In Figure 1-1, I've charted my real estate sales for the first eleven years of my career. When I first started, I was part-time and sold only three homes during the entire year. The number of sales grew each year, but a significant shift occurred in 2007 when I started sharing what I was doing with other real estate agents in my coaching group. Many whom I had helped were appreciative and went out of their way to find ways to help me in return. As they began sharing their ideas with me, my business took off!

It takes time to answer people's questions and to write about the things that are working or not working in your business. There is no immediate benefit for helping others except knowing that you helped someone stay in business and feed their family. Over time, the benefits of sharing become very apparent. I landed real estate accounts with six major banks because of introductions to key bank personnel by some of the "strangers" I'd helped online and later met at conferences!

Sharing has also helped me build amazing friendships with other positive-minded real estate agents in other states and provinces. By sharing best practices with one another, we've established a kinship and camaraderie that enables us to have fun while learning, sharing, and succeeding together.

Charitable institutions struggle in a tough economy, because the people they depend on are also struggling. I've heard many people say that they would give to charity if they ever became successful and wealthy. Unfortunately, that's not how it works. It's through *giving* that you experience success and wealth, so putting off giving is actually putting off your dream of becoming successful and wealthy!

CHAPTER 1 – BELIEVING IN ABUNDANCE

It's no coincidence that the most charitable people are also the most successful people. Look around your community. Those who give their time, talent, and financial resources to promote charitable causes have the most success. These leaders know the secret of the universe!

Your Beliefs Become Your Reality
When the economy takes a turn for the worse, fear of the unknown causes humans to hoard things. This happens most often when we allow the media or those around us to convince us that there is a scarcity of something. We store the information as a subconscious thought and it soon becomes entrenched as a belief. Since our beliefs control our actions, if we *believe* that a shortage exists, our actions will bring about the shortage, whether it is real or not!

Giving something away creates an opposite belief, that there is *abundance*. This information is also stored as a subconscious thought and also becomes a belief. The belief of abundance means that there is more than enough for everyone and that more will come to replace whatever we give away. If you possess this belief, your brain will be continually searching for opportunities to replace whatever was given without you consciously knowing that you're doing it!

By helping someone who has far more problems than you do, you can't help but feel fortunate. When your thoughts are consumed by feeling fortunate, you *become* fortunate because the belief that you are fortunate is driving all of your actions. But if you allow your thoughts to be filled with worry and fear, you will be so focused on avoiding danger that you won't see the opportunities that are right in front of you!

If you believe you have it tough, you will… If you worry about not having enough, you won't. Don't get caught in the trap of "poor me" self-pity. You will only find opportunity if you believe it exists. What you <u>think</u> about <u>comes</u> about. If you believe that you live in a world with an abundance of everything, you will have abundance. If you believe that you live in a country with more opportunity than any other place on the planet, you will find endless opportunities; they will present themselves. My mother put it best more than forty years ago when she told me, "You can't out-give God." Mom was right!

John Fox, a Life Success Coach in Tucson, AZ, is on a personal mission to educate everyone he meets about the secret of success outlined above. John's company, Think Out Loud Masterminds, offers a 10-week course that enables people from all walks of life to apply the principles from Napoleon Hill's book, <u>Think and Grow Rich</u>, in their every-day life.

John is passionate about helping people change their lives for the better. He moderates the 10-week sessions dozens of times a year and never charges for his class! John has helped hundreds if not thousands of people find success and happiness within themselves. Their success is his reward.

For ten weeks, I watched John draw a figure to illustrate how external events can affect our actions. I've recreated the

CHAPTER 1 – BELIEVING IN ABUNDANCE

diagram in Figure 1-2. For more information about John Fox and his life-changing class, go to: **www.tolmasterminds.com**. I highly recommend John, his course, and his company. He is an inspiration to everyone he meets.

Figure 1-2 How Events Affect Our Actions

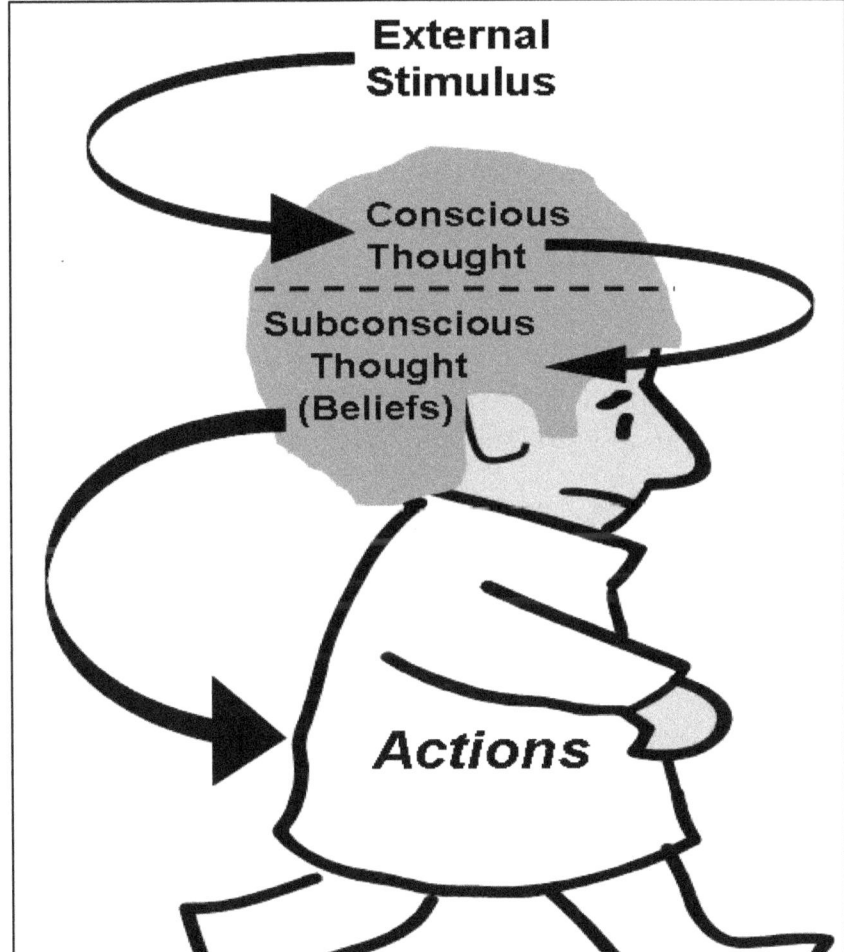

2

Fun with Flamingos

"We make a living by what we get, but we make a life by what we give."– Norman Macewan

A DAILY DIFFERENCE

Gena Foster in Jackson, Michigan, wanted to teach her 12-year old son, Chace, that sharing with others could be fun and rewarding. As a single parent and a real estate broker in a small town, she had limited resources but wanted to find a way to help those diagnosed with cancer in her community.

When Gena shared her desire to help, a friend told her about the fun they'd had raising money by putting up dozens of plastic flamingos in the yards of their unsuspecting friends. Curious, Gena did some research on the Internet and found information on two websites:

www.flamingofundraising.com
www.pinklawnflamingos.com

The websites provided step-by-step instructions of how to use the strange-looking birds to raise money. Intrigued, Gena ordered 30 of the large, hot pink, plastic birds. On the night the shipment arrived, Gena and Chace crept onto their neighbor's yard in the dark of night and installed the flamingos along with a yard sign with their company name that read, "You've Been FLOCKED!"

They had barely gotten the 30 flamingos in the ground when they saw the headlights of their neighbor's car coming down their quiet street. They ran to their home next door and watched in the dark from the windows as their neighbors pulled in their driveway and just sat in the car staring at the flamingos.

CHAPTER 2 – FUN WITH FLAMINGOS

When their friends finally got out of the car, they walked around the birds scratching their heads and finally decided to go inside. On the front door of their home, they found the notice shown in Figure 2-1 explaining that the flamingos were part of a fundraising effort.

Figure 2-1 You've Been FLOCKED! Notice

**Congratulations
You've Been Flocked!**

Don't Despair…
This is a fundraiser by Chace Properties for The Mission of Hope Cancer Fund.

A friend of yours paid us to place these pink darlings in your yard. This flocking is done in good spirits and is not meant to be mean. These flamingos will roost on your lawn until this evening when they will mysteriously migrate to another friend's (victim's) lawn.

If you would like to specify the next victim, all we ask is a small donation to our group.

Of course, the removal of these flamingos will be done at no charge, so please don't hurt our pink feathered friends.

Again, thank you for your sense of humor and your support.

Gina Foster
Chace Properties
(XXX) XXX-XXXX

Gena also provided their neighbors with a certificate for Anti-Flocking Insurance, shown in Figure 2-2. This "Insurance" provides protection from future flockings for only $10.00.

A DAILY DIFFERENCE

Besides offering to remove the birds free of charge if requested, their letter encouraged the "flocked" homeowners to "flock a friend!"

Figure 2-2 Anti-Flocking Insurance Certificate

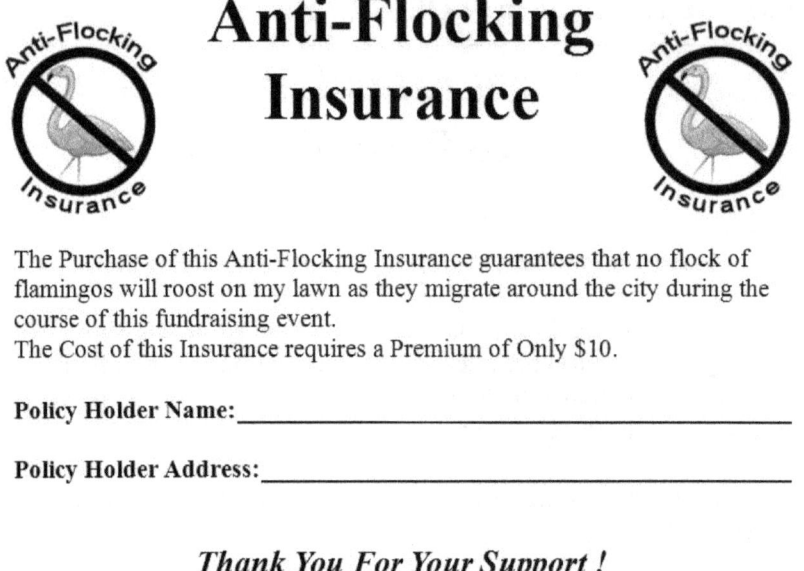

For $1 or so per bird, they will move the flamingos to the next victim's yard and repost the signs and paperwork. Each person flocked subsequently chooses the next victim to play a joke on and pays to move the birds.

After several minutes of uncontrollable laughter, Gena and Chace found their "flocked" neighbor at their door waving a twenty dollar bill excitedly. He said, "That is the funniest

CHAPTER 2 – FUN WITH FLAMINGOS

thing I've ever seen! Here's my money, you *have* to flock our friends!" A few minutes later Gena and Chace were driving down the road to their second flocking of the evening. This time the owners were at home.

The next morning, Gena found a posting on her Facebook wall from the woman they'd flocked at the second home. Apparently, at first glance that morning, her husband had thought the birds were eating all the grass seed he'd put down the day before! When Gena and Chace went to retrieve the flamingos, they found the notice still on the door of the home with a check stapled to it and a request that they flock the woman's sister.

Without having to ask for a penny, Gena and Chace had people practically throwing money at them for their charitable efforts and they were having a lot of fun raising the money together. In their first month of flocking, only one person did not pay to migrate the birds to another yard to "flock" a friend.

When they got their first order to flock the home of someone they didn't know, Chace asked Gena what they would do if they were caught. Without much thought, Gena replied, "How can you be mad at someone with their hands full of plastic flamingos?"

Sometimes they are caught in the act of flocking. When it happens, they make the people who caught them help to flock one of their friend's homes. They've picked up several volunteer flockers along the way who move the birds when Gena has other commitments.

A DAILY DIFFERENCE

On one such occasion, Gena's friend, Hannah, flocked a local pastor's yard. The next day, Gena received a call from Hannah wondering if she had retrieved the birds from the pastor's home. Gena didn't know where the birds had been deployed and was very upset. *Who would steal thirty pink flamingos from a pastor's yard?*

Gena posted an All Points Bulletin on Facebook for her flamingos, asking anyone who saw them to notify her of their location. She then began driving up and down every street in the area until she found the birds in someone's yard. After finding nobody home, Gena didn't know what else to do so she called the police. When the policemen were done laughing at her, they agreed to send an officer over to "investigate."

Shortly after her awkward conversation with the police, an SUV full of giggling teenage girls pulled into the driveway of the "flamingoed" home. The conversation got off to a rocky start, but Gena calmed down and explained that the flamingos were generating revenue for the Mission of Hope Cancer Fund and that she was teaching her son that helping others can be rewarding and fun. It turned out that the girls were members of the high school golf team and had "borrowed" the flamingos to play a prank on one of their unsuspecting teammates.

Soon, a police officer showed up and the girls became visibly nervous. Gena told the girls that since they'd proven their ability to move the flamingos to their friend's yard, a proper punishment for "borrowing" the birds would be to take responsibility for moving them for the next two weeks. The

CHAPTER 2 – FUN WITH FLAMINGOS

girls quickly agreed, relieved at not being charged with thirty counts of "flamingo filching."

A month later, I saw Gena at a real estate conference in Dallas. She told me that the girls on the golf team were having so much fun flocking people that they wouldn't return her flamingos. Gena has a contagious passion for helping others and it was a shame that her fundraising ambitions were being limited by a flamingo shortage. When I found out that the flamingos had cost less than $6 apiece, I gave her the money to buy another flock. I'd sold several copies of my books at the conference and had a pocketful of money to help her.

While shopping for replacement birds, Gena found them on sale and was able to buy TWO flocks of flamingos with the money I'd given her. The girls on the golf team had become Gena's first flocking franchise and her friend, Hannah, became the second franchisee. With the infusion of flamingos, Gena's efforts could be tripled every day, but she didn't stop there…

When her assistant's daughter was stationed in Afghanistan, Gena and her team decided to offer their flocking services to families with loved ones overseas in the military.

For a small donation they'll send soldiers two dozen pink flamingo suckers, a pair of crazy flamingo sunglasses, a Bible, and a pink card that reads, "YOU'VE BEEN FLOCKED". The text on the back of the pocket-sized card is provided in Figure 2-3.

A DAILY DIFFERENCE

Figure 2-3 Soldier's Pocket Card

> A thousand may fall at your side,
> ten thousand at your right hand,
> but it will not come near you.
> You will only observe with your eyes
> and see the punishment of the wicked."
> Psalms 91:7-8
>
> We are the people of his pasture,
> the FLOCK under his care.
> Psalm 95:7

In their first six months of flocking, this single mom and her twelve-year-old son raised nearly $3,000 for the Mission of Hope Cancer Fund. Their selfless efforts have provided many cancer patients in their community with assistance to cover medical equipment, prescriptions, insurance premiums, transportation costs to and from treatments, housing costs for out-of-town treatments, and additional medical costs. For more information about the Mission of Hope Cancer Fund go to: **www.cancerfund.org.**

One of the recipients of their flocking revenue is the family of Miley Pickell, a three-year-old who has T-cell Lymphoblastic Lymphoma. Miley has spent far too much of her young life undergoing treatments but has an unstoppable spirit. A photo of Miley is on the front cover of this book and in Figure 2-4.

CHAPTER 2 – FUN WITH FLAMINGOS

Figure 2-4 Miley Pickell

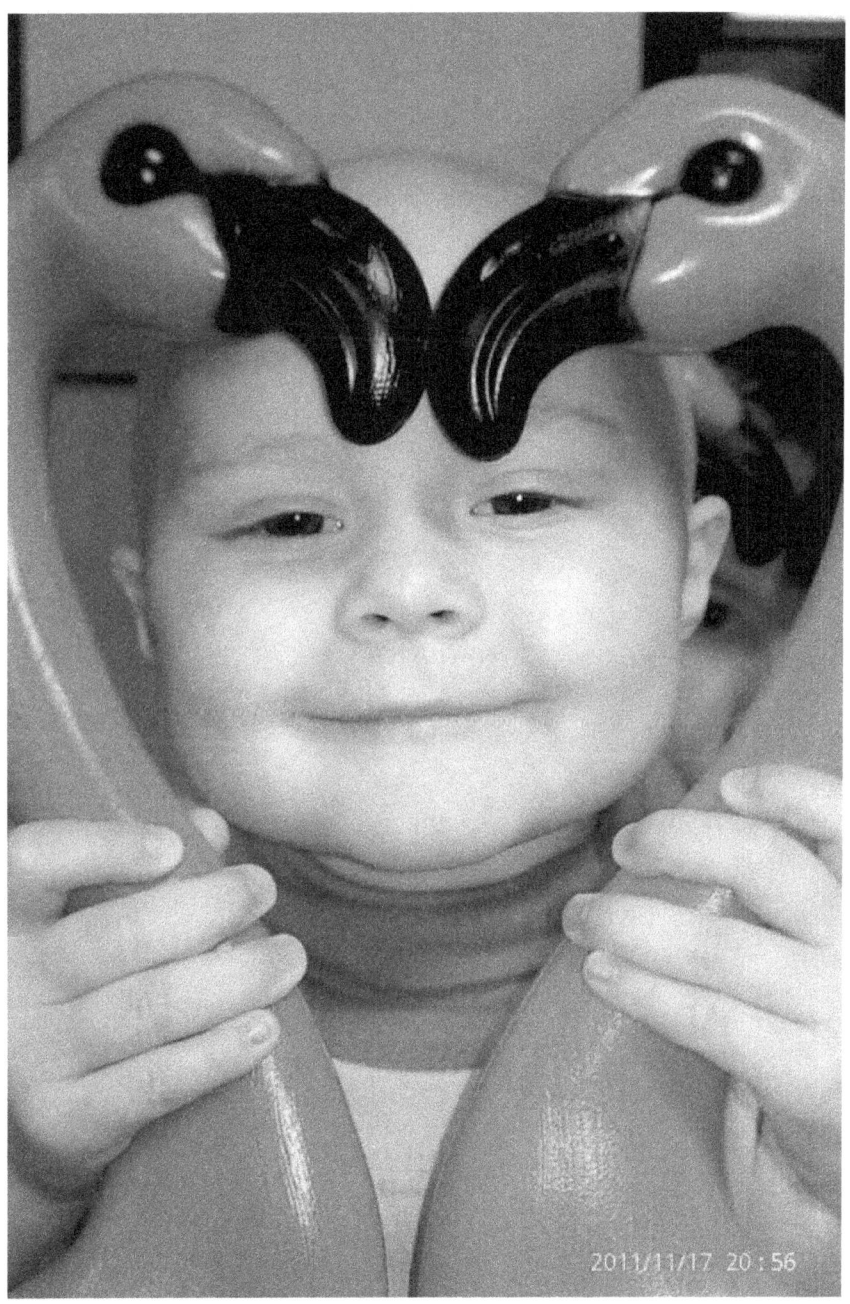

A DAILY DIFFERENCE

Although Gena did not invent flocking, her contagious passion has spawned three flocks of revenue-producing flamingos and an international mission to amuse and protect soldiers. Through their selfless acts, Gena and Chace have inspired people they've never met thousands of miles away. They are making a difference in their community and in the world. I am proud to call Gena my friend and appreciate her sharing this story with me so I could share it with you. Get Flocking!

3

Cookies For Campers

"When it comes to giving, some people stop at nothing."
– Anonymous

A DAILY DIFFERENCE

For six years, my wife, Camille, and I served on the Board of Directors of Montlure, a Christian children's camp in the White Mountains near Greer, Arizona. The camp is nestled on 10 acres in the Apache-Sitgreaves National Forest, which boasts the largest continuous stand of Ponderosa pine trees in the world. At about 7,000 feet elevation, the temperature at the camp is usually 30 degrees cooler than either Phoenix or Tucson.

Besides donations, the camp's only source of revenue was eight weeks of summer camp during June and July. We were always searching for other ways to raise money. There are limits to how often a non-profit group can tap their donor base to ask for money, so you really need to make each contact count. Choosing a fundraiser is one of the most important decisions a charitable group must make throughout the year.

In 2002, the Board of Directors decided to sell frozen cookie dough to fund needed repairs at the camp. Since I had a flexible work schedule, I volunteered to meet the delivery truck to receive the Tucson allotment of cookie dough. On a warm Tuesday in July, it quickly became apparent that the timing of the cookie dough campaign hadn't been well thought out. As the delivery truck driver and I unloaded hundreds of tubs of the frozen dough into our 100 degree garage, I began to wonder how we would keep it all cold.

After filling our refrigerator, both freezers, and every ice chest we owned, I went to one of our vacant rental homes to remove the shelves in the refrigerator and stack it and the freezer with cases of the quickly-thawing dough. We

CHAPTER 3 – COOKIES FOR CAMPERS

frantically called every telephone number we had for the other cookie dough captains, but some told us that they would not be able to retrieve their cookie dough until Saturday. By then it would be cookie soup!

After much pleading and five days of driving to outlying areas, we finally had all the cookie dough delivered, picked up, or eaten. I'm certain that if we cleaned out our freezer today we'd still find a tub or two of petrified dough.

Across the state, the camp's supporters sold 350 tubs of cookie dough. At a price of $10.00 per tub, we grossed $3,500. In the minds of the people who bought the cookie dough, they'd given $10.00 to the camp, but Montlure received only $2.00 from every tub of cookie dough that was sold. When you consider the effort and gasoline involved in coordinating, selling, and delivering the cookie dough, the "profit" of $700 was not even enough to break even!

It disturbed me that only 20% of the money raised actually went to the church camp. This is something I've considered before embarking on any fundraising effort since then. In hindsight, instead of selling 350 tubs of cookie dough we could have earned more money for the camp by setting up a flock of 30 flamingos 23 times. It would have been a lot less stressful, a lot more fun, and a whole lot easier on everyone's waistline.

After the initial expense to buy the birds, every penny would have gone toward supporting the camp, instead of supporting the cookie dough company. The flamingos could

A DAILY DIFFERENCE

continue to raise revenue throughout the year because the plastic flamingos can't be eaten and they don't melt!

Since our fundraising effort didn't produce enough profit to finance any of the needed repair projects, we embarked on a grass-roots campaign to make people aware of the needs at the camp. Montlure has affected the lives of thousands since 1926, but was really showing its age. The number of campers had been declining each year and so did the allocation of funds for preventive maintenance. In short, the camp was headed full-throttle into a death spiral.

With another summer camping season fast approaching, we scheduled several work weekends at Montlure to get the winterized camp operational. Our small, twenty-family church at Tortolita Presbyterian in Tucson gathered a group of ambitious volunteers to make the 180 mile trek on the first work weekend. Upon arriving, many of the volunteers couldn't believe how dilapidated the camp had become.

The electrical service had been spliced many times and the underground lines were exposed in some places. Luckily, one of the volunteer members of our work party that weekend happened to own an electrical contracting company in Tucson. Ron Gamble was known in our church for giving regularly of his time and financial resources. He was always one of the first to volunteer for church projects.

After inspecting the camp's electrical system, Ron got on the phone and started ordering some things that were needed. The more he explored the more phone calls he made.

CHAPTER 3 – COOKIES FOR CAMPERS

During each of the next three work weekends, Ron and his four man crew accompanied Harold and Hazel Copenhaver, Todd and Kathy Dirkschneider, and Camille and I to the camp with truckloads of materials and heavy equipment. They rewired the entire facility with new service panels, wiring, and light fixtures. Ron's generosity inspired the rest of the congregation to donate appliances, cabinets, flooring, paint, and a variety of other materials. After only a month, the camp was literally transformed!

With the updated electrical service and other generously donated improvements, Montlure was safe, clean, and ready for campers. We spent much of the summer writing and updating more than 250 processes and procedures for camp operations. In July, Montlure was inspected by the American Camping Association and was certified as a safe and well-run camp.

With improved facilities and ACA certification, Montlure began to attract more campers. The revenue from the additional campers was used to add new programming and hire a year-round manager to promote and care for the camp. The work camps continued during the off-season and within three years, the number of kids attending camp had more than tripled! The newly found revenue provided even more programs and improvements.

It's humbling to walk around the camp and realize that every nail, board, and hour of labor to construct the twenty-plus buildings was donated by ordinary people. The camp represents generations of passionate people who gave freely of

A DAILY DIFFERENCE

their time, talent, and financial resources to improve the lives of children. It's scary to think of how close we came to losing that peaceful, serene place and the tens of thousands of hours lovingly spent to create it.

I learned several things from this experience:

1) The follow-up after a gift is just as important as the gift itself. It does no good to give someone a car unless you also provide them with some money for gasoline. Before a new building is constructed, 10% of the building's cost should be allocated in the budget each year to maintain it.

2) Situations don't change by themselves. Change occurs when someone has a vision, shares it with others, and motivates them with their selfless effort. Showing others what to do always works better than *telling* them what to do.

3) A small number of dedicated people focused on the same goal and inspired by a leader can overcome a seemingly impossible task. More than 100 churches send their kids to Montlure, but one of the smallest congregations came forward to save it, giving more than all of the other churches combined that year.

Unfortunately, this ratio is all too common in our society. Even though we have all benefitted in some way from the gifts of others, only a small minority give their time and financial resources for the greater good of the community. Whether donated parks or Little League coaches, generations of adults have made the effort to improve children's lives.

CHAPTER 3 – COOKIES FOR CAMPERS

The next time you see someone volunteering, stop whatever you are doing and offer to help them. It will change your world and theirs!

In recent years, several other churches in the state have stepped forward to support and fund Montlure. Unfortunately, in June, 2011, the camp was right in the middle of the Wallow fire, the largest forest fire in Arizona history. Although the surrounding mountainside was entirely blackened for miles, thanks to the diligent efforts of firefighters, only five buildings at Montlure were lost in the fire. On aerial views of the area, Montlure looks like a golf green in a sea of charred forest.

It will take years to stop the erosion, replace the buildings, and reopen the camp, but many who have a place in their heart for Montlure are rallying their forces to overcome this latest obstacle. Go to **www.montlure.org** for information about how you can help. There may be some frozen cookie dough in it for you!

4

A Blue Öyster Birthday

"There is no delight in owning anything unshared." – Seneca

A DAILY DIFFERENCE

In 2009, with my 50th birthday fast-approaching, I didn't have a mid-life crisis or try to compensate the way many adult males do. I decided to forego getting a Harley Davidson or Corvette and celebrate what I hoped would be the half-way point of my life by raising money for the Make-A-Wish Foundation. Since I was turning 50, I set a goal of raising $50,000.

I chose Blue Öyster Cult, a 70's rock band, to perform at my fundraising event. I'd seen the band perform live at Texas Jam in the Houston Astrodome thirty years earlier. Their hit song, "Don't Fear the Reaper," seemed a perfect way to celebrate fifty years of adventurous living. The marketing poster created to promote the event is provided in Figure 4-1.

As you might expect, hiring a famous band can be quite expensive, even if the peak of their fame was three decades earlier. After calculating the cost of the band and the venues at which they could perform, I decided to hold a "Business Builder" real estate training event to raise the money. I hoped that sharing the things that had enabled us to sell 500 homes that year would encourage other real estate agents from across the country to attend.

Every well-laid plan has its surprises and I experienced more than a few in this venture. Who knew that the cost of constructing the stage, installing the lights, and renting the instruments would total more than $12,000? The promotion company was another $5,000, but due to the charitable nature of our event, the promoter reduced the rate to $2,500 and two hotel rooms.

CHAPTER 4 – A BLUE ÖYSTER BIRTHDAY

Figure 4-1 Blue Öyster Cult poster

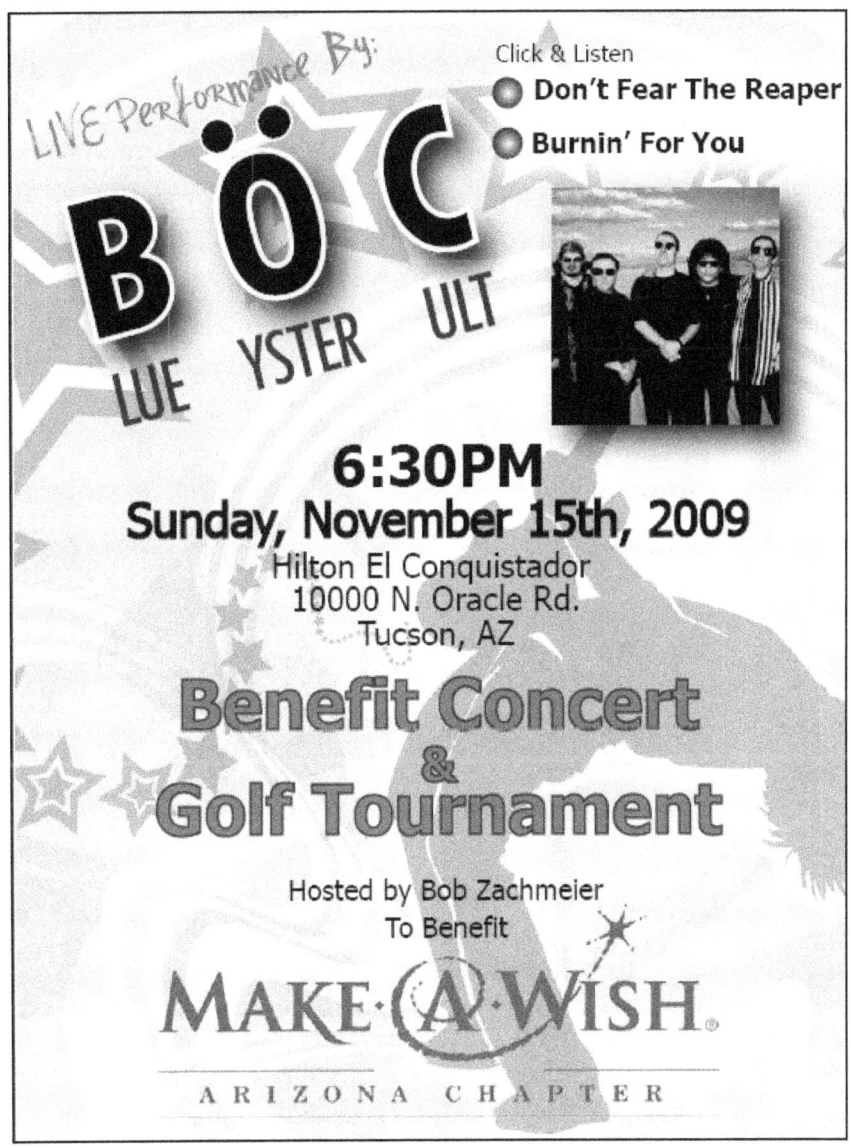

An on-call limousine service and seven additional hotel rooms for the band were not in my budget either so I had to

A DAILY DIFFERENCE

find creative ways to raise even more money. To offset these unexpected costs we offered golf tournament sponsorships and backstage passes to meet the band prior to the show.

Many of my top-producing real estate agent friends came to the rescue by purchasing backstage passes, or simply making donations. Tom and Naomi Moon paid for a sponsorship and brought two staff members with them from Huntington Beach, CA, to support us. A backstage photo of Blue Öyster Cult and the friends who helped pay for the unexpected expenses is provided in Figure 4-2.

Figure 4-2 Blue Öyster Cult Backstage

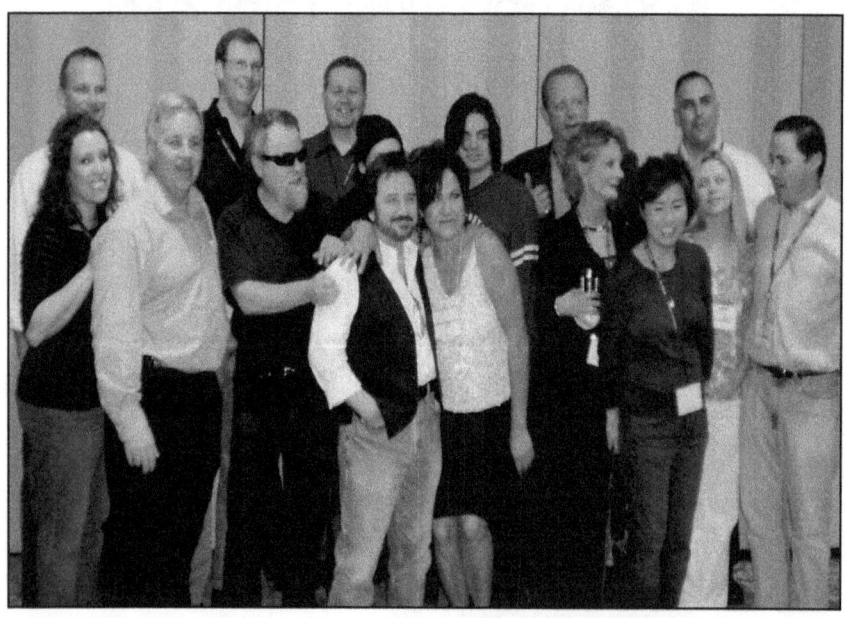

Back Row: Scott Miller, Ed Laine, Adrian Petrila, Danny Miranda (BÖC), Jules Radino (BÖC), Lester Cox, Jared Erfle **Front Row:** Amy Coleman, Bob Zachmeier, Eric Bloom (BÖC), Buck Dharma (BÖC), Carmen Rodriguez (from my office), Pat Cox, Victoria Erfle, Julie Reekie, Ian Reekie **Not pictured:** Tom and Naomi Moon, Aaron Kinn, Chase Horner, David Connart, Igor Krasnoperov, Steven Blackwood, Teresa Ryan, and Ray Valle

CHAPTER 4 – A BLUE ÖYSTER BIRTHDAY

One day after a real estate closing, I was relaying my unexpected budget discrepancies with the ladies at Stewart Title. I'd worked with this escrow team for more than ten years and they asked if they could help by conducting a silent auction at the event. They could see that I was overwhelmed with all the other aspects of the event, so they asked only for a list of the vendors our company had utilized in the past.

Using only the QuickBooks list I'd given them, they contacted each vendor to ask for items to include in the silent auction. On the day of the event, I was in awe at the quantity and quality of the items they'd collected, packaged, framed, and inventoried. I will be forever grateful to Joann Bersell, Debbie Turner, Kim Moss, Catherine Alameda, Julie Benson, Lauren Duffy, and Tori Bentley. In addition to the hundreds of hours they logged before the event, they also conducted the silent auction and collected the funds from each winning bidder.

When we counted the proceeds at the end of the night, I was shocked to find that without any help from me, they'd raised $13,500 with the silent auction! Your friends can accomplish a lot when they find out you need help. All you have to do is make them aware of the need and get out of the way!

When I met Eric Bloom, the lead vocalist of Blue Öyster Cult, before the concert backstage, he asked if I appreciated the discount he'd given me for the event. I apologized and explained that I'd never hired a major band before and had no idea how much they normally charged for a performance.

A DAILY DIFFERENCE

Eric informed me that after the Make-A-Wish Foundation began in Phoenix, Arizona, a lady in New York wrote a letter to the editor of the New York Times suggesting that they start a chapter there. Eric responded to the woman and together, they founded the Make-A-Wish chapter in New York State. How cool is that? I guess letters to the editor work!

When Eric learned that our event was benefitting the Make-A-Wish Foundation in Arizona, he discounted the band's rate by $20,000! A photo of Eric Bloom (left), Buck Dharma (right), and Jules Radino (drums) is provided in Figure 4-3.

Figure 4-3 Blue Öyster Cult Concert photo

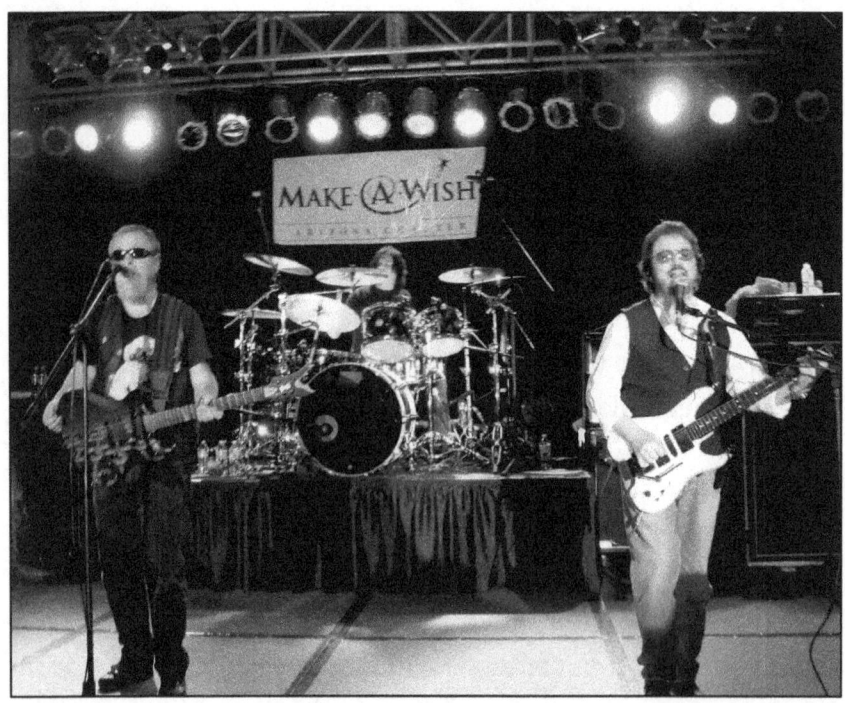

CHAPTER 4 – A BLUE ÖYSTER BIRTHDAY

Without the help of my friends who purchased the backstage passes and sponsorships, the ladies at Stewart Title Company, everyone who supported the silent auction, and Eric Bloom and the members of Blue Öyster Cult, the unforeseen expenses would have caused my fundraising event to be a fund-losing event. Instead, through many acts of kindness, we raised over $27,000 for the Make-A-Wish Foundation that night. When combined with the $100 we donated for every foreclosed home we sold throughout the year, we surpassed the seemingly unachievable goal of $50,000. To see a video from the event, go to **www.vimeo.com/8255175**.

It seems that some things are just meant to be. No matter how many challenges you face, if you stay focused on the goal, involve your friends, devise creative solutions, and keep working toward the end, your dream will become a reality!

All of the unexpected expenses from the Blue Öyster Cult fundraiser forced me to find other ways to raise money. The "Business Builder" real estate training class I created was very well received and several people who attended told other real estate agents about it. Soon, people began asking when I would hold another class.

We no longer offer headliner bands, but have expanded the course content. Each event now includes two full days of "in the trenches" training to share how we've adapted our company to meet the challenges in the ever-changing real estate market. Attendees of the conference make their checks

A DAILY DIFFERENCE

payable to whatever charity we are supporting to help needy kids in our community.

Since 2009, these "Business Builder" events have become a semi-annual event to help others in the agent community and underprivileged kids in our community. Besides bringing business to local hotels and restaurants, we've also generated more than $100,000 for children's charities in Tucson.

For information about upcoming "Business Builder" training events, please e-mail: **event@win3realty.com**.

5

Caring Kids

"There are three ways to get something done: do it yourself, employ someone, or forbid your children to do it."
– Monta Crane

A DAILY DIFFERENCE

Through my work with the Make-A-Wish Foundation®, I've had the privilege of meeting two former "Wish Kids." Although these "kids", now teenagers, face life-threatening health problems, both Lizzie Bell and Camden Garcia have chosen to focus on helping other kids rather than spending their time worrying about themselves.

Lizzie Bell

Lizzie is one of only 700 people in the world with Diamond Blackfan Anemia, a condition in which the bone marrow produces an insufficient number of red blood cells. As a result, she requires a blood transfusion every few weeks. Her wish was to swim with the dolphins in Hawaii.

During one of Lizzie's bi-weekly visits to the hospital, she overheard a nurse telling a little boy who was struggling during a procedure that he would receive a toy after they were finished. Imagine the disappointment the little boy experienced when he later lifted the lid of the toy box and found that all the toys had been given away.

When Lizzie witnessed that event, she wanted to make sure that it wouldn't happen again. She created Lizzie's Loot™ and actively recruits toy donations for hospitalized kids coping with a life-threatening medical condition. Her program has brought joy to thousands of hospitalized kids each year by ensuring that they have something to look forward to after each visit to the hospital for a potentially uncomfortable procedure. The photo in Figure 5-1 was taken at the benefit concert held in Tucson on my 50th birthday.

CHAPTER 5 – CARING KIDS

Figure 5-1 Lizzie Bell and Bob Zachmeier

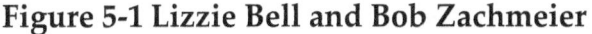

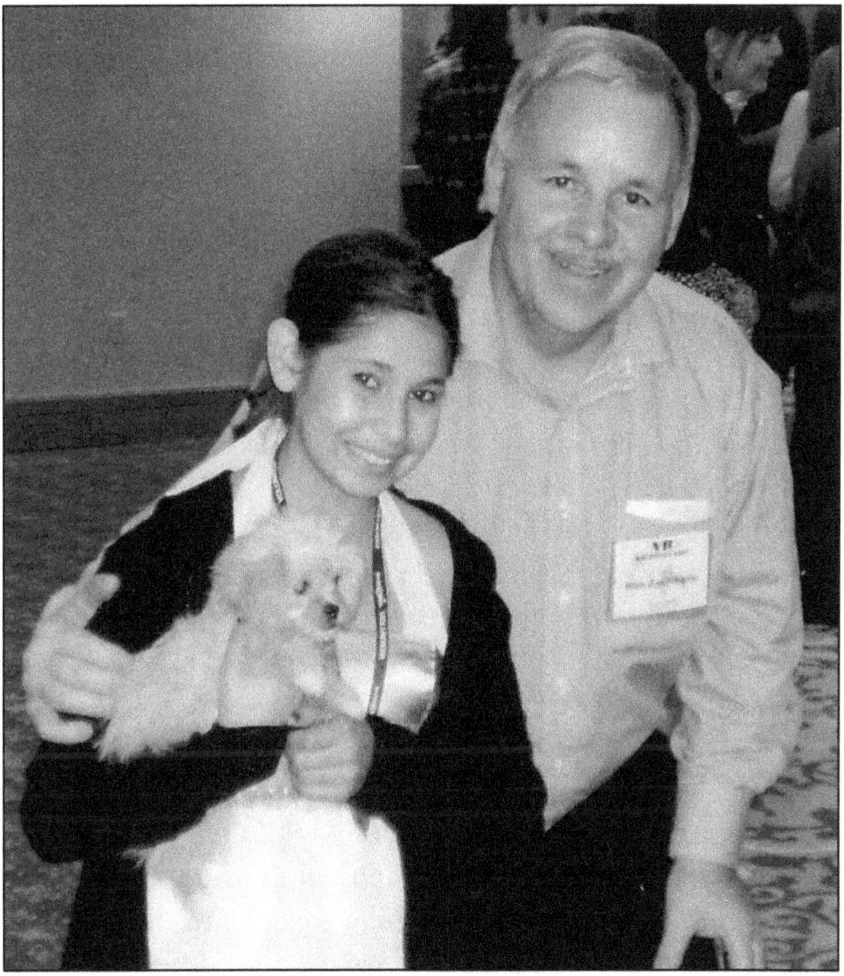

Besides her passion for keeping toy boxes filled, Lizzie has also become a regular spokesperson for blood donation awareness and the National Marrow Registry. She tells anyone who will listen about the importance of donating blood and it is working! More than 12,000 pints of blood have been donated in Lizzie Bell's name since she began her campaign in 2010.

A DAILY DIFFERENCE

Lizzie is also an ambassador for the Red Cross and was inducted into the Blood Donor Hall of Fame! Her passion for making a difference has attracted the attention of national celebrities like Miley Cyrus.

Lizzie did all this even though she must check into Diamond Children's Hospital every other weekend for 72 hours of medication! Below are some quotes from Lizzie's website, **www.lizziebell.org:**

I'm alive because of people like you who continue to donate blood. But I'm not the only child in need of blood. There are many children who depend on blood donations because of burns, injuries, surgeries and more. Just one pint of blood donated from an adult will save up to three lives. You can help by donating blood at your local blood donation center. Every 2 seconds someone needs blood or blood products.

You may have seen me last year on the ABC Television Program, "Extreme Makeover - Home Edition". My family was chosen to receive a new house. It's beautiful! Our old house was falling apart and our new home was built in about 100 hours. It was awesome! More than 3,000 volunteers participated. It's amazing what we can do when we work together.

Spending so much time in hospitals during the past 15 years has given me a clear view of the things that kids need to make them more comfortable and less fearful while they're in the hospital for treatment.

CHAPTER 5 – CARING KIDS

Send me an email if you need more information about how and where to make tax deductible contributions to my foundation (John P. Bell Family Foundation) to help us fund our projects for kids, or if you'd like more information about the television program "Extreme Makeover", if you'd like more information about donating blood, or if you just want to talk to me, personally. I answer all of my emails and I'd be delighted to talk to you.

We update our website with new information, events and campaigns, so come back and visit here often. You'll find lists of things that are happening, places where I've been invited to speak, Fund Drives, Blood Drives (in your area) and more. But you can help kids like me right now - today. When you contribute funds or blood, you help medically fragile kids like me get through another day.

Camden Garcia

Camden is an inspiring teenager who is wise beyond his years. At the age of five he developed a brain tumor which caused a series of seizures and other serious complications. To help his family deal with the long series of treatments and impending surgery, Camden was chosen as a "wish kid" by the Make-A-Wish Foundation®.

Camden's wish of attending a NASCAR race and meeting Jeff Gordon, his favorite driver, was fulfilled when the entire family was picked up in a limousine and flown to Fort Worth, TX. After three days in an owner's box at Texas Motor Speedway and a private tour of Jeff Gordon's pit, they returned with a lifetime of memories and a variety of merchandise personally autographed by Jeff Gordon.

A DAILY DIFFERENCE

Camden has been cancer-free for over ten years, but that experience gave him the desire to help others in a similar situation. Camden's father, Gil, and mother, Carol, own Kustom Steel, a metal fabrication company that makes steel security doors and other products in Tucson, Arizona.

After many years of working with his father in their shop, Camden has become an accomplished welder. He takes the scraps punched from the metal and other hardware and welds them together into crucifixes. From spark plugs to diamond-shaped metal scraps, he artfully welds together what some would refer to as "junk" and creates a masterpiece.

Camden sells his completed crucifixes and donates the profits to the Make-A-Wish Foundation®. His crosses have sold at auctions for as much as $1,400 apiece. At a recent "Business Builder" training event we held in Tucson, Camden earned more than $3,600 for the Make-A-Wish Foundation from his crosses.

Camden has given back far more than the cost of the wish he was granted but continues to support the organization that made such an impact on his family when they were going through a difficult time. To find out more about Camden and his mission to help others, go to **www.camdenscrosses.com**. You can purchase his crosses online.

We all have a skill, talent, or knowledge that has value to someone else. You may have to be creative to find a way to utilize your expertise, but if everyone worked as hard at helping others as Lizzie and Camden, the world would be a

CHAPTER 5 – CARING KIDS

much better place! Figure 5-2 is a photo of Camden with one of the crucifixes he creates.

Figure 5-2 Camden Garcia

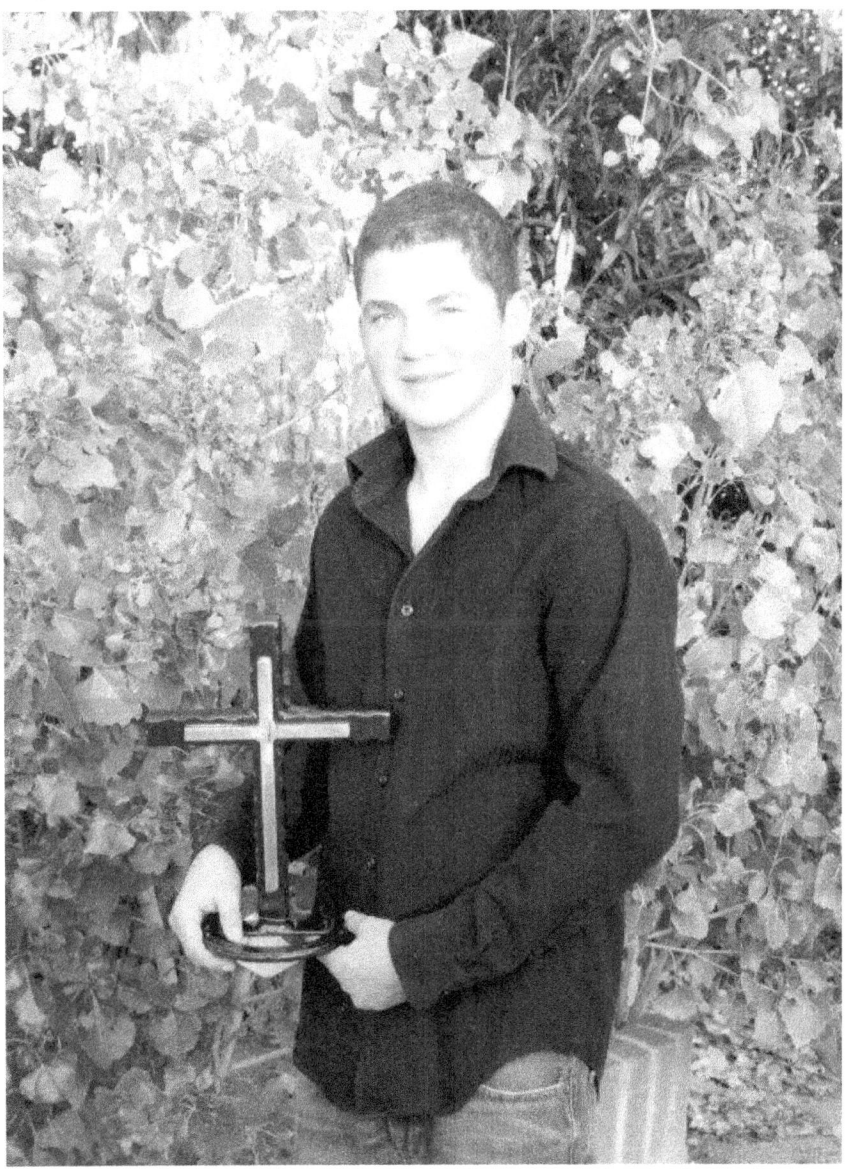

A DAILY DIFFERENCE

If two young teens with medical challenges can make such a tremendous difference in their community, why can't you? Isn't it strange how the people who need help the most are the ones who *give* the most?

Their health issues make most of the "problems" others face in life seem irrelevant and trivial. Follow the example of these inspiring young people and find a way to "pay it forward" to someone else! To find out more about the Make-A-Wish Foundation go to **www.wish.org**.

6

Power in Numbers

"The test of our progress is not whether we add more to the abundance of those who have much; it is whether we provide enough for those who have too little."– Franklin D. Roosevelt

A DAILY DIFFERENCE

I've gotten to know many top-producing real estate agents across the United States and Canada through Craig Proctor's real estate coaching program and the REObroker.com broker network founded by Tom Moon. All of the real estate agents who helped to defray the unexpected expenses of my birthday fundraiser are from these two groups. We've known one another for several years, but my birthday event was not the first time we came together for charity.

In May, 2009, eleven of us pooled our resources to raise money for the Make-A-Wish Foundation at the National REO Brokers Association (NRBA) conference. Besides the charity auction at their annual conference, NRBA members are asked to pledge $100 from every real estate closing in the month of July to the Make-A-Wish Foundation. We all signed up to do so, but took it one step further. What if we shared $100 from EVERY closing throughout the year?

Our group of top-producing real estate agents began sharing best practices with each other and coordinated client visits to several lenders throughout the country for whom we sold foreclosed properties. None of us knew at the time that we had laid the foundation for what would become a not-for-profit organization called Real Estate Organization for Kids, or REO4Kids. A copy of our marketing flyer is provided in Figure 6-1.

We decided to make REO4Kids a not-for-profit group rather than a non-profit to avoid unnecessary overhead. The donations we collect are paid directly to the charities we support so there is no question about where the money goes.

CHAPTER 6 – POWER IN NUMBERS

Figure 6-1 REO4Kids Marketing Flyer

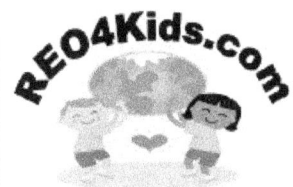

WHO WE ARE

Our Leaders
We're a goodwill epidemic that's rapidly spreading across the country. We support children's charities by donating our time, talent, and money to those less fortunate. We serve our local and national communities by providing outreach programs, training, fundraising activities, and by giving a $100 donation for real estate transactions we close. Our network is growing as the word spreads about how a focused consistent effort can make a difference in the lives of thousands.

Our Vision
We envision a future made brighter by improving the lives of children today.

Our Mission
To enable children, especially those who need the most help, to reach their full potential as our next generation of adult leaders.

Our Goal
Our goal is to improve the future of children in need in our communities across the nation. Our long-term goal is to provide children in need the opportunity to obtain a good education, show others what hard work and endurance can accomplish, and lead a successful life of sharing in the communities they live in.

Our Strength
Our strength is in our numbers. As we add new members across the nation, the amount of time, talent, and financial resources donated to children in need will also increase. Our HOPE is that the spread of good will toward local children will heighten the awareness of those in need and inspire others in our communities to open their hearts to help those around them.

Pay It Forward!
Real Estate Organization 4 Kids
www.REO4Kids.com

REO4Kids collects $500 in annual dues from each member to offset marketing expenses and fees for exhibition booths at real estate conferences to further our cause. A photo of the REO4Kids exhibitor booth is provided in Figure 6-2.

Figure 6-2 REO4Kids Exhibitor Booth

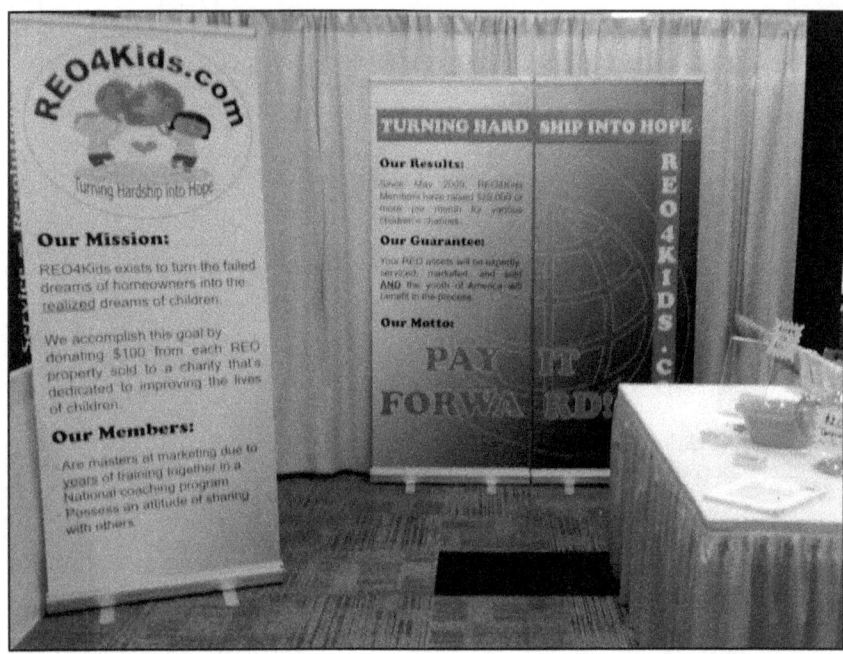

In 2009, the 11 members of REO4Kids sold more than 2,000 homes and donated more than $200,000 to the Make-A-Wish Foundation®. Because foreclosures were having such an adverse affect on inner city kids, in 2010, REO4Kids adopted Boys & Girls Clubs of America and began donating $100 for each foreclosed property we sold. During the first three months of 2010, our small group of 18 real estate agents raised an amazing $67,000 for children's charities.

CHAPTER 6 – POWER IN NUMBERS

We were well on our way to achieving our annual goal of $250,000 when I had the idea of asking the financial institutions we worked for to *match* our contributions. If we were giving $100 to charity maybe they could too! Within a few hours of making the request, Ken Blevins, the CEO of PMH Financial in Denver, Colorado, agreed to do it! The gift from PMH Financial received national attention. A copy of the article in REO Insider magazine is provided in Figure 6-3.

Figure 6-3 REO Insider Article

REO4Kids Aims to Raise $250,000 for Charity in 2010
PMH Financial, which provides financial services and asset management, agreed to match member donations from the nonprofit REO4Kids to the Boys and Girls Club of America.

Every time an REO property sells with the 18 nationwide members of REO4Kids, a $100 donation is made to the Boys and Girls Club of America. REO4Kids launched a year ago, and since then, the group has been trying to recruit asset management firms like PMH and other financial institutions to match the donation on sales of their REO properties. The group raised $67,000 in Q110 and hopes to donate $250,000 by the end of the year.

Bob Zachmeier, broker and owner with Win3 Realty in Tucson, Ariz., and a participator in REO4Kids, said if the targeted lenders and servicing companies contributed like PMH, they could exceed $500,000 in donations this year. Zachmeier added that it costs $500 per child to provide after school programs for one year.

"If we are able to double our goal, we'd be able to keep 1,000 at-risk kids off the streets and would save many lives," Zachmeier said.

In May, 2009, a group of 11 REO brokers and agents attending the coaching services for the National REO Brokers Association (NRBA) agreed to pool their resources and good will to start REO4Kids. In 2009, REO4Kids raised money for the Make-A-Wish Foundation.

In November, 2009, the group of agents swelled to 18. Members write quarterly checks to Boys and Girls Club of America, setting aside the donations monthly.

A DAILY DIFFERENCE

If all of our clients would be as generous as PMH Financial, we could *double* the $250,000 goal we'd set that year. PMH Financial also matches the funds their employees raise each month for local charities. They have an amazing corporate culture that attracts some really fantastic people.

There is magic in numbers. When a group of one hundred people all focus on the same goal, amazing things can happen. If one member raises or donates $100 and the effort is matched by the other 99 people in the group, $10,000 is raised for the charity. If each volunteer raises $1,000, then the charity receives $100,000. We determined that if we could recruit 100 members to the group and raise an average of $10,000 per member, we could give a million dollars *every year!*

The magic works in reverse with expenses. To pay a $100 bill, each person need only contribute *one dollar!* There is no other way I've found to *multiply* your income and *divide* your expenses by one hundred! The best part is that nearly half of the amount contributed comes back to those who donate it as a tax refund.

Since forming REO4Kids in May, 2009, we've grown the membership and donations each year. No matter what you do or how much you earn, EVERYONE has something to share. It takes time and effort to explain a new process or campaign, but if you share an idea, shortcut, or process with other people, most will feel obliged to find a way to pay you back.

When people offer to pay me for the help I've given them, I gladly accept and ask them to make their check payable

CHAPTER 6 – POWER IN NUMBERS

to the Make-A-Wish Foundation® or Boys and Girls Club. This allows my sharing to make an impact on the person I helped and also on the kids supported by my two favorite charitable causes.

When you share information, you win by knowing that you did something to help, the person you helped wins because their business improves, and the charity wins by receiving more funding. If you can find a way to turn everything you do into a win-win-win situation like this, you can't help but succeed in business and in life.

The more you help people succeed, the more they will have to share with others. The more people receive help, the more they want to provide help, so the initial gift is passed on and on into infinity. The two "wish kids" featured in Chapter 5 are a perfect example of how a gift can continue giving.

REO4Kids members meet several times per year at real estate conferences, but the power of the group is the daily sharing on an e-mail chat line. If someone in the group has a new advertising campaign or sign they want to try out, they send an email to other members in the group with their idea, success, or request for help. It's uncommon to have a problem posted that someone in the group has not already experienced in their market. On most requests for help, several solutions are posted within a matter of hours or even minutes.

Several members of our group are the top-selling agent in their state and almost all are in the top ten in their local markets. What value would you place on the ability to tap the

A DAILY DIFFERENCE

best minds in your industry on a daily basis? There are coaching programs charging tens of thousands per year that don't come close to providing the amount or quality of materials that our members share with each other on a daily basis.

REO4Kids is *not* for takers! When new members are considered, we look for more than just real estate sales. We seek out successful people who are involved in their community. People who have a passion for giving are prone to give more than they take from our group. We also conduct a background check and require proof of donations, not because we don't trust our members, but because we want to share innovative new ways to raise money with the rest of the group.

Membership in REO4Kids is growing as we attract new "givers," to the group, but real estate commissions have declined drastically in many areas and some members are not able to contribute as much as they have in the past. In 2011, our company 67 homes that paid $1,000 or less in commission, which doesn't come close to covering our costs.

Rather than stopping our charitable giving, we've had to find creative ways to *raise* the money rather than donate it. Chapters 7 through 13 contain innovative ways that other members of REO4Kids have found to raise money in a challenging economy to improve the lives of children. For more information about REO4Kids and a current list of its members, go to **www.REO4Kids.com**.

7

Change From Lunch

"You must give to get, you must sow the seed, before you can reap the harvest." – Scott Reed

A DAILY DIFFERENCE

In a world where many people take more than they give, Amy Coleman, of Sacramento, California, is an anomaly. Because she was always one of the biggest sharers in our coaching group, I immediately recognized her name when I met her for the first time at a conference.

Amy was always helping other agents by sharing every success and tidbit of information she acquired with the members of our coaching group. We immediately formed what would become a lifelong friendship. What I appreciate most about Amy is that she doesn't just *talk* about things, she <u>does</u> them! When we were forming REO4Kids, she drafted the By-Laws on the plane ride home from the meeting and sent them out for the other members to review when her plane touched down.

Ever since we founded REO4Kids, Amy has been a member of the Executive Board of Directors and the group "Mom" to all members. We don't call her that because she coddles everyone; it's because she holds members accountable for their actions and their commitments to deadlines. Amy is actually one of the youngest members of the group, but her youthful energy and constant nudging has kept the group moving forward. The world is full of good intentions, but success requires leadership. Amy Coleman has made an awesome contribution in that regard.

Amy's business partner, Bruce Hammer is also passionate about helping children. Having been orphaned at the age of five, Bruce has personally experienced the negative effect that an environment without traditional family support

CHAPTER 7 – CHANGE FROM LUNCH

or parental figures can have on kids. Without some redirection in his life, or meals and clothing from the parents of friends, Bruce's life might have turned out dramatically different, as it did for many of his peers.

Bruce is appreciative of those who helped him when he needed it and is constantly looking for opportunities to give back. He knows that his charitable giving and physical support to children's charities will help to ensure a positive future for generations of children who otherwise might not have the chance or desire to succeed in life.

Together, Bruce and Amy own Golden State Realty, Inc. in Sacramento, CA. The housing downturn hit California hard with daily news reports about mortgage defaults, foreclosures and evictions. The real victims of a housing downturn are the children, who in many cases no longer have their yard, their room, or their friends. Amy and Bruce use their real estate company to raise awareness of the plight of these children and more importantly, to get others they meet to help out financially.

Whether speaking at conferences, agent training events, meetings, or simply going over options with a new client, Amy and Bruce use the opportunity to educate people about the needs of these kids. They've learned that word-of-mouth can be a tremendous fundraising opportunity so they preach from the proverbial mountaintop for all to hear. They have been known to match the donations of clients who support children's charities like the Make-A-Wish Foundation® and Boys and Girls Clubs.

A DAILY DIFFERENCE

Some people may think that helping others and giving back to your community is difficult or time-consuming but to Bruce and Amy it can be as easy as serving food at a homeless shelter or donating old clothes, food, or money to worthy organizations. Bruce and Amy are on a mission to help those who, due to a variety of circumstances, are unable to help themselves.

Something as simple as donating pocket change can affect many lives if more than one person is involved in the effort. When a group of people come together to make a difference, other people are inspired to help. Sacramento is a city of nearly a half million people. If each person donated just two dollars per *year*, nearly a million dollars could be raised to help needy children.

Amy and Bruce decided to make a difference, one house at a time, by donating a portion of each real estate commission they earn. Due to their regular giving, they developed a heightened awareness that has led to other "out of the box" ideas for raising funds to help local children-centric organizations. *What you think about comes about!*

While returning home from a conference, Bruce was thumbing through the Skymall catalog and found a company selling six-foot-tall, standing advertising banners. The ad gave Amy the idea of creating a banner for their office conference room that would serve as a visual aid for raising donations. In a collaborative effort, they designed a banner that states "Help us help KIDS… Change from Lunch can Change a Life" A photo of the banner is provided in Figure 7-1.

CHAPTER 7 – CHANGE FROM LUNCH

Figure 7-1 Conference Room Banner

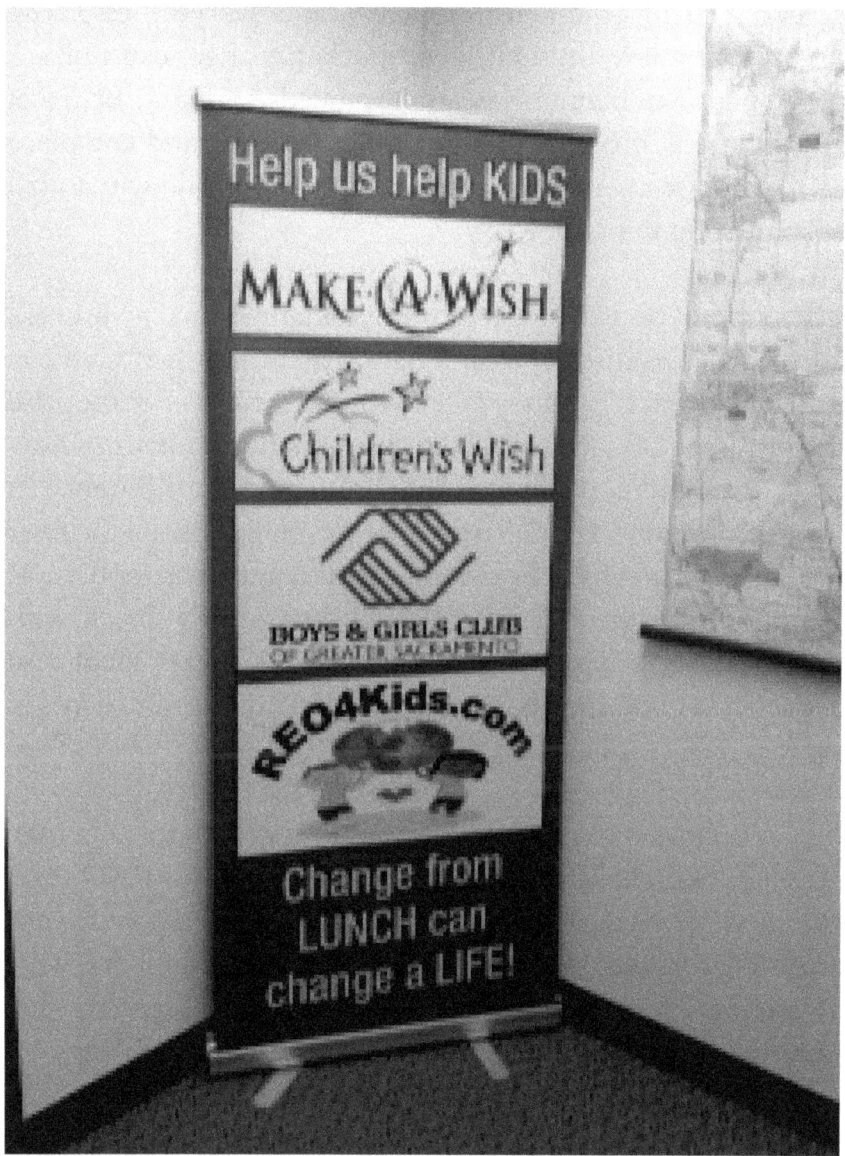

A DAILY DIFFERENCE

The banner is a reminder to friends, family, clients, potential clients, their cleaning crew, and everyone else who sees it that every little bit, even pocket change, can make a difference. The banner has accompanied Amy and Bruce at presentations, office meetings, training classes, and any place they can raise awareness. There is no more certain way to fail at something than not to try.

Amy and Bruce also implemented an awareness campaign to educate their clients that they can make a difference, too. When they meet with potential clients, they use the last page of her PowerPoint presentation to discuss how their company and other clients are making a difference in their community. They also give their clients a copy of the flyer in Figure 7-2 that lists the charities their company supports. At the bottom of the flyer is a dotted outline of a check with "Attach Check Here" in bold lettering. You get what you expect in life and they have convinced many of their clients to write a check for children's charities!

Besides making them aware of easy ways to help, they activate their client's Reticular Activator System (RAS). You may be asking yourself, "What is a RAS?" Well, everyone has one. RAS is the part of your brain that heightens your awareness of certain things. For example, if a person just purchased a new car, on the drive home they will have a heightened awareness of all the other cars like theirs on the road. The same number of cars like theirs were probably on the road on their way to the dealership, but they didn't notice them because they had no reason to isolate them from other cars.

CHAPTER 7 – CHANGE FROM LUNCH

Figure 7-2 Client Donation Flyer

Donation to Children's Charity

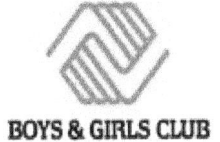

Near and dear to our heart's ♥ is helping children.

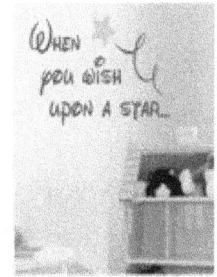

Share the Power of a Wish.

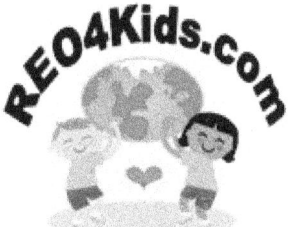

We regularly donate to these children's charities to help make a difference in our local communities.

BONUS: You get a tax write off!

 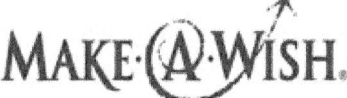

Attach Check Here
Payable to:
Boys & Girls Clubs of America
or
Make a Wish

A DAILY DIFFERENCE

So what does a RAS have to do with giving to charity? Amy and Bruce introduce the topic of giving to get those around them thinking about making a difference by donating time, money, clothing, or food to charities. This simple awareness campaign can change thousands of lives. By adding one slide to their presentation, they have raised thousands of dollars, from a handful of pocket change to donations of one hundred dollars or more.

After promoting charitable giving all year, Amy and Bruce planned a big surprise for a local charity on December 24, 2011. Through their efforts, they'd been able to raise and donate $4,500 to the Sacramento Boys and Girls Club. They were pleased that their fundraising had gone so well and were excited about being able to give the Club their check on Christmas Eve.

Unfortunately, their excitement was deflated when they opened the morning newspaper to find that Wells Fargo had donated $30,000 to the Boys and Girls Club the previous day. Amy and Bruce still delivered their check as planned, but they walked into the Club with their heads hung low. They presented their "measly" $4,500 check stating, "We know it isn't that much but here are a few dollars we raised for your club."

With shrieks of joy and overwhelming excitement, the Chapter CEO called her entire staff into her office to show them the check. She introduced Amy and Bruce to everyone and praised the two shocked agents for helping to change children's lives. Her reaction rejuvenated the excitement in

CHAPTER 7 – CHANGE FROM LUNCH

Amy and Bruce. They realized that although their small company couldn't compete with large corporate donors, every bit helps and is appreciated. Bruce said, "That $4,500 check could have been a million dollars in the eyes of the club employees. It was such an exciting and rewarding feeling to be able to make a difference in people's lives."

The power of numbers is how this world will change. It all starts by activating someone's RAS to get them thinking about how they can help. Everyone can make a difference, one person at a time. Giving back to your community is as simple as the acronym "GIVE."

Gratitude – Be thankful for what you have and notice others who have much less. Show others how they can help you to make a difference.

Investment – Spend your time and energy in addition to or in place of money. There are endless ways to help, so find one that utilizes your skills and talent.

Volunteerism – Offer your time. Get friends and family members to join you. Helping others can be a great family outing and much more rewarding than other activities.

Encouragement – Encourage others to make a difference. Through education and awareness you can activate other people's desire to take action.

A DAILY DIFFERENCE

Change from lunch really can change lives! To find out more about Amy Coleman and Bruce Hammer and the innovative ways they are helping the kids in their community, go to: **www.sacramentohousefinder.com.**

8

Everyone Can Do Something

"The more sympathy you give, the less you need."
– Malcolm Stevenson Forbes

A DAILY DIFFERENCE

Lester Cox is a founding member of REO4Kids and has served on the Executive Board of Directors since the inception of the group in 2009. Lester grew up in Kansas City, Missouri, but his family relocated to Arizona after his father died when he was 17. Lester inherited his father's strong work ethic and the belief that there is no ceiling on what a person can achieve.

As the oldest member of REO4Kids, Lester has assumed the role of a father figure for the group. He is relied upon to be the voice of reason to resolve disputes and to use his experience to provide practical solutions to other member's problems. During his 40 years in real estate, Lester has sold more than 5,000 homes and is one of the few people to reach more than a billion dollars in sales. He willingly shares his experience and is well-respected in the industry.

Lester and his wife of 37 years, Patricia, have strived to help disadvantaged and at-risk youth for more than thirty years. They own and operate Pacific Arizona Realty in Tempe, AZ. Besides running their real estate brokerage, Lester spends a good part of each day helping others become successful. He is a professional real estate coach for Craig Proctor Coaching and facilitates two mastermind groups.

As a member of the National REO Brokers Association, Lester serves as the Master Broker for Arizona. He is responsible for coordinating the annual fundraising effort for the Make-A-Wish Foundation® and helping other members improve their business.

CHAPTER 8 – EVERYONE CAN DO SOMETHING

I could go on and on about all of the things Lester does on a day-to-day basis, but I've learned that if you ever need something done, *give it to a busy person*. Lester's favorite quote is from Mother Teresa, who once said, "Never worry about the number of people needing help. Help one person at a time, and always start with the person nearest you." In the Arizona real estate market, you don't have to look far to find someone who needs help.

The Arizona Department of Education reported that more than 29,600 homeless children were enrolled in public schools in 2010, a 21% increase from the previous year and a 160% increase from 2003. With so many foreclosures, mortgage defaults, and evictions happening in our cities, the number of displaced families and children is growing at an alarming rate.

Patricia says, "Whenever I enter a foreclosed property, the first thing that strikes me are the things left behind – I am quickly reminded that a child has lost their home. Not only have these children had to bear their parents' stress through financial hardship, they no longer have their familiar bedroom, yard, or neighborhood playmates. How terrible this must be for these little folks."

Operating under the assumption that, "Nobody can do everything, but everyone can do something," Lester and Patricia served on the original Board of Directors of Valley Big Sisters long before Big Brothers and Big Sisters were combined. Before the merger, Big Sisters had no corporate sponsors - just a group of hard-working volunteers who wanted to make a difference in the lives of young girls. By providing strong and

A DAILY DIFFERENCE

enduring one-on-one relationships, these dedicated volunteers helped hundreds of young girls realize their potential.

The group was almost fully funded by the efforts of the Board members, so money was always very tight. The group not only survived in their dingy old building downtown, they grew due to the leadership of the Executive Director, Linda Searfoss, who had a lot of talent and a huge heart. Most Board meetings centered on how to make the next payroll.

The group's biggest fundraisers were organizing and running casino nights and golf tournaments which would sometimes raise as much as $5,000 in an evening. That was really big money at the time, but the amount of work was enormous. All the gaming equipment had to be rented, picked up and assembled, dealer volunteers had to be trained on the various games, scripts had to be printed, and bars had to be stocked. The biggest and hardest task was getting prizes donated and tickets to the event sold. Each volunteer would spend days of preparation to ensure the success of each event.

Their efforts were all worthwhile when the results of each little girl's successes were relayed to the group by the big sister, the little sister, or the director. Today the unified Valley Big Brothers and Big Sisters organization is the oldest, largest, and most effective youth mentoring organization in the United States. Research has shown that positive relationships between "Littles" and their "Bigs" have a direct and measurable impact on children's lives. They are more confident in school, better able to get along with their families and peers, and less likely to begin using alcohol and drugs.

CHAPTER 8 – EVERYONE CAN DO SOMETHING

Lester and Patricia never had children of their own, but they have been blessed with many nieces and nephews and now grand nieces and grand nephews that are all like their own kids. For the most part, their "kids" are all healthy and well. They have all learned to give back by observing and helping Lester and Patricia over the years.

One of their favorite activities was volunteering to deliver dinners to homes of needy families on Thanksgiving. There was a restaurant owner in Phoenix, Arizona who would collect money throughout the year and then also donate all the food and labor to cook the Thanksgiving dinners; in fact, he would close his business the day before and Thanksgiving Day just to prepare the meals.

Lester and Patricia would arrive at his restaurant around 5:00 AM to load their van with all the Thanksgiving fare. Then they would deliver the meals to anyone who had asked for help. One year, they talked their 15 year-old nephew, Scott Graff, into going with them. Getting a 15 year-old up at 4:30 in the morning was not easy, but he did it and was extremely helpful.

Scott had been raised in a loving family and had never wanted for anything, but all day long he was able to see and meet many less fortunate people. That day he learned to appreciate his parents for the lifestyle they'd provided but also, through Lester and Patricia's actions, he learned to never turn his back on anyone whom he could help.

A DAILY DIFFERENCE

Lester and Patricia are also avid supporters of the Boys and Girls Club. In fact, Lester arranged a meeting in 2010 with REO4Kids members and both the chairman and national marketing director of the Boys and Girls Clubs of America. This meeting did an awesome job of raising our awareness about the plight of inner-city kids. Here are some statistics:

- 3 out of 10 kids in America won't graduate on time
- 15.1 million kids are unsupervised between 3 to 7 PM
- 3 out of 10 kids are obese or overweight
- 1 out of 5 kids live in poverty

Several members, including me, began supporting their local Boys and Girls Clubs after that meeting. We learned that the Boys and Girls Clubs of America has a mentoring program to train local leaders. Since many REO4Kids members had benefitted greatly from real estate coaching, it seemed like a natural fit to support the Boys and Girls Club's mentoring program.

We decided to contribute 20% of the funds we raised or donated to the national mentoring program and 80% to the local chapters in our communities. By sharing his passion for helping kids in the Boys and Girls Club, Lester influenced the decision of more than a dozen top-selling real estate agents to become involved in their local communities. It pays to share your passion with others! To find a Boys and Girls Club in your area go to **www.bgca.org**. To follow the charitable efforts of Lester and Patricia Cox go to **www.wesellaz.com**.

9

Follow The Leader

"Let your heart feel for the afflictions and distress of everyone, and let your hand give in proportion to your purse."
– George Washington

A DAILY DIFFERENCE

Teresa Ryan, of Naperville, Illinois, is one of the most compassionate people I know. She and her large real estate team contribute to over 90 different charitable organizations involving the care of animals, the planet, children, families, veterans, and just about anyone else in need.

As the owner of Ryan Hill Realty, Teresa and her husband, Nick, have built a unique team culture where their staff and agents all subscribe to their philosophy of giving back to the local, national, and international community. They are not just real estate agents selling homes; they are a family of dedicated people committed to making a positive impact on the lives they touch.

When their team decides to support something, they infuse the time, energy, and money to accomplish whatever challenge they face. The owners, agents, and staff all spend personal time on a variety of volunteer commitments in their community. Below are some examples of how an organized effort and an inspiring leader can make a huge impact:

Naperville Responds for Hurricane Katrina
When Hurricane Katrina struck the gulf coast, Teresa and Nick were horrified over the plight of the people in its path. They contributed $25,000 to launch a relief fund to help those affected by this disaster. With long-time Naperville mayor, George Pradel, and other compassionate community leaders, they formed a charitable group called "Naperville Responds" to help the victims of disasters, veterans, and other groups needing assistance.

CHAPTER 9 – FOLLOW THE LEADER

The real estate agents at Ryan Hill Realty followed suit by volunteering to contribute $50 from every closing in 2007. They ended the year with 380 homes sold and Ryan Hill Realty matched their contribution dollar for dollar, raising another $38,000. To date, their company and employees have raised or donated over $83,000 for disaster relief along the Gulf Coast. The funds help build homes in the devastated areas of the Gulf Coast through donations of building materials and monies donated by Naperville businesses and citizens.

Teresa's team doesn't just write a check and forget about it; they put butts on planes and boots on the ground! In January, 2008, <u>twenty</u> Ryan Hill agents and management flew to Pass Christian, Mississippi to join with the Mennonite Community to re-build a home for a family that had become homeless due to the hurricane. Their team members installed insulation and drywall, dug trenches, poured concrete, cleaned up, and hauled garbage as they bonded to help someone less fortunate.

They returned home with sore muscles from days of hard labor, but their enthusiasm and commitment made them return again in February, 2009, to help build another home for a homeless family. Teresa credits Bill Brestal, of Dommermuth, Brestal, Cobine & West, now retired, for leading this wonderful project. In all, Naperville Responds for Hurricane Katrina raised over *$2 million dollars* and built, with the guidance of the Mennonites, 21 homes in Pass Christian, Mississippi. A photo of Teresa and Nick Ryan working in Mississippi is provided in Figure 9-1. Nick is far left, Teresa third from right.

Figure 9-1 Ryan Hill Team in Mississippi

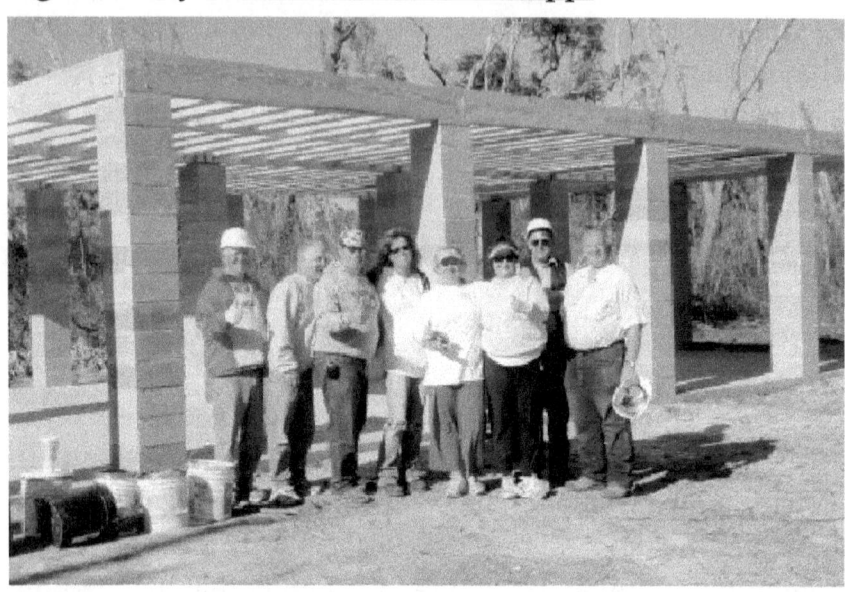

Naperville Responds for our Veterans

Appreciating what our veterans have endured for our country, Ryan Hill Realty helped to form a group of volunteers to assist wounded and disabled veterans returning from Afghanistan and Iraq by offering housing at little or no cost to them. Ryan Hill Realty team members have served on the Board of Directors, committees, and in the trenches helping veterans since the 501(c)(3) group was founded in 2009.

Since its inception, the program has assisted veterans from the Korean Conflict, World War II, Iraq, and Afghanistan with home repairs and updates. Recently they installed a wheel chair ramp for a veteran from WWII. The rewards are many for the community and the veterans who have sacrificed for our freedom. To find out more about Naperville Responds For Our Veterans, go to: **www.nrfov.com**.

CHAPTER 9 – FOLLOW THE LEADER

In 2009, the group started a campaign to gather and send letters, greeting cards, and photographs to military personnel deployed overseas, especially in war zones like Afghanistan and Iraq. Serving as a collection site, the company annually receives approximately 3,000 greeting cards and letters addressed to "American Hero." In 2009, over 5,000 cards were delivered. Everyone appreciates mail, especially when away from home in a hostile area over the holidays.

Children

Teresa believes that it is our responsibility to raise a generation that leads, enhances, and progresses. The children of this generation have evolved intellectually, with an astounding potential as a future society. There are also children who don't have choices, are orphaned or have special needs. To help them secure a better future, she contributes personally to over 20 organizations involved in improving the lives of children.

Beginning in 2008, Ryan Hill Realty partnered with Welch Elementary School to host 2nd grade students and chaperones at their company headquarters for their annual field trip. Students learned about the careers available in real estate as well as other types of businesses.

During the past four years, over 400 children from the 2nd grade class have visited Ryan Hill Realty. Each year, the agents on Teresa's team return the favor by visiting the 2nd grade students and teachers at their school. A photo of the second graders visiting Ryan Hill Realty is provided in Figure 9-2.

Figure 9-2 Teresa Ryan with Second Grade Class

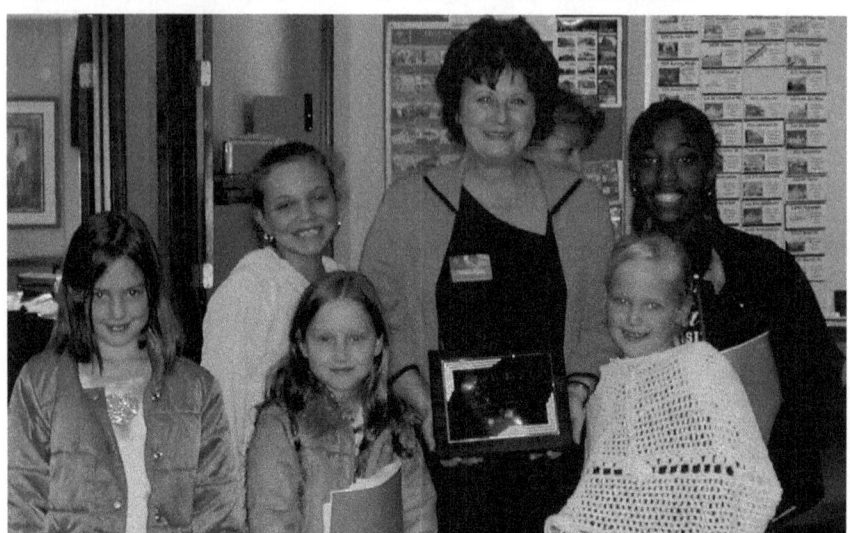

Animals

Due to the nature of the real estate business, Teresa often finds abandoned pets in the homes they inspect. Some of the more unique finds were a cockatiel and two clown fish! The fish were in a tank and had survived for more than a month without care. All creatures great and small are valuable to Teresa, and she ensures that all rescues are placed in the best care and good homes.

By enhancing the quality of life for those around them, Teresa Ryan's real estate team has created an improved environment in which to do business and live. Their passion for helping others can be seen throughout their company

CHAPTER 9 – FOLLOW THE LEADER

because everyone has a sense of personal involvement and group fulfillment that propels them to take on new challenges with a "can-do" spirit that breeds success.

For example, each month, someone on Teresa's team volunteers to assist the overnight mission in neighboring Aurora, Illinois. The work involves opening the doors at the mission at 7:00 PM, feeding and caring for 150 people, including children and families, and providing them with a place to sleep. They are fed again at 7:00 in the morning to get their day started.

Teresa chose an office in the heart of downtown Naperville to be involved in every aspect of her community. From Easter egg hunts to Saint Patrick's Day parades, high school athletes to Special Olympics coaching, Teresa and her team are involved or leading. Through their charitable efforts, they've developed instant recognition and ever-growing trust throughout their community. A company culture like this is difficult to find, but it can be reproduced. All it takes is one person to care enough to make a difference. Leaders are followed and Teresa Ryan leads with passion!

For more information about Teresa Ryan and the Ryan Hill Realty team go to: **www.ryanhillrealty.com.**

10

Creative Fundraising

"A bone to the dog is not charity. Charity is the bone shared with the dog, when you are just as hungry as the dog."
– Jack London

A DAILY DIFFERENCE

Nancy Braun owns Showcase Realty in Charlotte, North Carolina, where she has been a real estate agent for sixteen years. Prior to owning a real estate brokerage, Nancy was an attorney and chef/restaurant owner. Nancy is one of the most creative fund raisers I know. She has shared some of her creative ideas in this chapter.

Agent Training and REO4Kids

In 2010, Nancy joined Reo4Kids and was inspired to step up her charitable efforts so she began contributing to the Boys and Girls Clubs of Charlotte. She was simultaneously awarded a contract to sell homes for the Department of Housing and Urban Development (HUD). A requirement of being a HUD listing broker is to hold monthly workshops for real estate agents to educate them about selling HUD homes.

Nancy decided to hold the monthly workshops at a Boys and Girls Clubs facility so she could use the opportunity to not only educate the real estate agents about HUD homes but also about the efforts and mission of the Boys and Girls Clubs of Charlotte. While she doesn't charge for these workshops, she asks the agents to make a donation to the Club if they feel so inclined.

Nancy allows affiliated businesses such as title companies, lenders, and home inspectors to participate in the training and speak briefly to the group in exchange for a donation to the Boys and Girls Club. These affiliates donate prizes for raffles and make it fun for the agents who attend. Nancy provides the required training to the real estate agents, the affiliated businesses receive the opportunity to speak with

CHAPTER 10 – CREATIVE FUNDRAISING

the agents, and the Boys and Girls Clubs receives donations from Nancy, the affiliates and the agents, a win-win-win situation. In 2011, Nancy raised over $4,000 for the Boys and Girls Clubs of Charlotte from the workshops she is *required* to hold! She also made a contribution for each property she sold.

As a result of Nancy's generosity, she was asked to join the Boys and Girls Clubs of Charlotte Advisory Council. She is also on the Marketing Committee and is Chairperson of Resource Development for the Club. Nancy is responsible for overseeing the three most significant fundraising campaigns the Club conducts during the year. Since becoming involved with Boys and Girls Clubs she learned:
- 57% of alumni say that "the Club saved my life"
- 67% of all children graduate high school in 4 years
- 93% of 2-year Club members graduate in 4 years
- 97% of 4-year Club members graduate in 4 years

Clearly this program works and Nancy is proud to be a part of it! For more information about the Boys and Girls Clubs go to **www.bgca.org**. To watch a video about the Charlotte Club, go to: **www.youtube.com/watch?v=J9g8O3No97o**.

Basketball Player's Furnishings

Nancy was assigned a foreclosed home that had previously belonged to a retired NBA basketball player. The home was nicely furnished so Nancy contacted the former owner and found that he didn't want the furniture left behind. Typically the bank hires contractors to haul away the personal property, but Nancy asked if she could hold a yard sale. The bank declined her offer due to the potential liability involved.

A DAILY DIFFERENCE

Determined not to let the expensive furnishings be thrown away, Nancy received permission from the bank to have a consignment shop pick up most of the furniture. The Salvation Army came and took the rest. She negotiated with the consignment shop to give the Boys and Girls club 60% of the proceeds and made fun price tags for each piece so potential purchasers would know that most of the proceeds were going to a good cause.

The bank saved money by not having to hire someone to remove the furniture, the Salvation Army gave the remaining furniture to a family who needed it, and the checks are still coming in for the Boys and Girls Club whenever another piece of consigned furniture is sold! For information about the Salvation Army, go to: **www.salvationarmyusa.org.**

Dog Rescue

As a real estate broker, Nancy has helped many families going through foreclosure in recent years. She is especially sympathetic to the innocent victims of foreclosure, the children and animals.

One situation left a lasting impression on her. At a foreclosed home she found two dogs that had been left outside without any cover. The smaller black dog was locked in a tiny cage with knee-high feces that had not been removed for weeks. The dog had cleared a little space to sit by pushing her feces into a pile at the rear of the cage. The other dog, a blonde chow, was on a chain that had become imbedded in his neck.

CHAPTER 10 – CREATIVE FUNDRAISING

Neither dog had been socialized so Nancy was a bit afraid, but feeling sorry for them, she bought a huge bag of dog food and some raw meat which they quickly devoured. Both dogs were starving, so she went to the property and fed them daily while trying to find another place for them to stay. Afraid to call animal control because she was certain that the animals would be euthanized, Nancy made arrangements to transport the dogs to the home of a friend who had kennels and the space to keep them.

After cleaning the dogs, she took them to a veterinarian and found that the little black dog had been repeatedly impregnated and both dogs had heartworm. Treating the dogs for heartworm would cost over $2,000 and would take 6 weeks. Since the treatment involves arsenic, the dogs can't move around a lot or the arsenic could get into other parts of their bodies and kill them.

Nancy paid for the heartworm treatments, spaying, neutering, shots, and the dog's food and supplies while they were being treated. She cared for the dogs during the six weeks and they became socialized and learned how to walk on a leash. They turned out to be great dogs; all they needed was to be loved and cared for. After the waiting period following the heartworm treatment, Nancy was able to convince the Humane Society to take the now healthy dogs (and her $1,000 donation to the shelter).

Shortly after arriving at the Humane Society, Kelly, the chow was adopted and a few months later Samantha, the scared little black dog was adopted. A photo of Kelly (left) and Samantha (right) are provided in Figure 10-1.

Figure 10-1 Kelly and Samantha

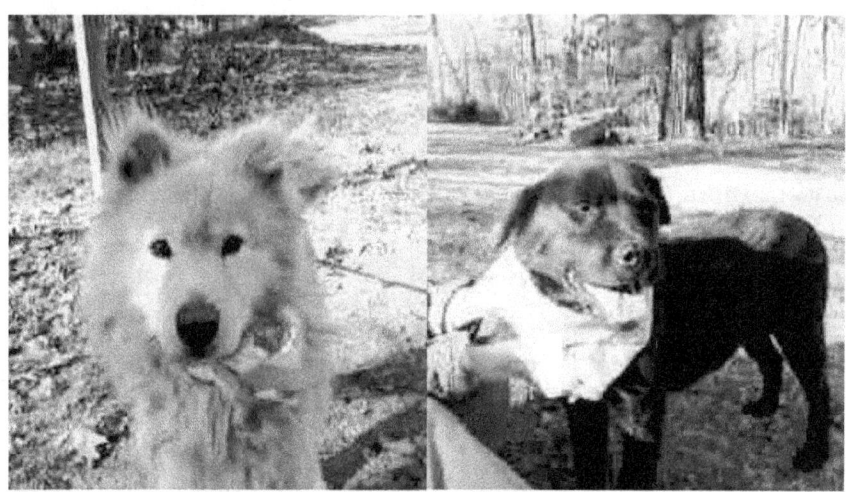

Nancy says she feels like she was selected to sell foreclosed homes so she could rescue the animals victimized by foreclosure. In this case, she saved two dogs that otherwise would have suffered a different fate.

In these situations, Nancy's creativity and passion made a huge difference. Her donations and unique ideas resulted in more than $22,000 being given to local children's charities in 2011. In a slow real estate market, Nancy increased her charitable contributions and her business became more prosperous. Giving and receiving seem to coincide with one another; all you need is a passion for making a difference and a creative mind. For more information about Nancy Braun, go to: **www.showcaserealty.net**.

11

Leaving Footprints

"If you haven't got any charity in your heart, you have the worst kind of heart trouble." – Bob Hope

A DAILY DIFFERENCE

Pat Koch, a real estate agent in San Diego, California, has been an advocate of children for most of her adult life. She and her husband, Bernie, had a life-changing experience in October, 1999, while on vacation in Jamaica. They had taken time away to celebrate Bernie's birthday at a resort in a quaint fishing village. During their stay, they became friends with other vacationers at the resort and agreed to meet them the following year during the same week.

When they ventured into the village away from the resort areas, Pat was dismayed at the poverty they found. They toured the elementary school in Duncan and were shocked to find that most of the children had no shoes, limited teaching materials, and the facilities were hideous. Pat was heartbroken over how these children had nothing. They had been born into poverty and had no way of getting out, especially if they didn't have a chance of getting a decent education.

Pat, Bernie, and several of the friends they'd met at the resort decided to improve the situation for these children. They created a Children of Jamaica trust fund and raised funds to purchase teaching equipment which included TVs, VCRs, DVD players, books, and even a freezer. They also created a website where they posted the footprints of all the children who needed shoes.

For more than a decade, their travel to Jamaica became an annual event during the same week every October. Each year, their group became bigger as they met new people. The group now includes people from all over the United States and

CHAPTER 11 – LEAVING FOOTPRINTS

Canada who have joined their crusade to help the local children.

With the help of the resort, their idea caught on with other regular guests who visit the resort during different weeks of the year. Soon Pay Less Shoes became involved and began donating hundreds of pairs of shoes each year. Before long, all the school children had at least one pair of sturdy shoes, so the group shifted their focus to providing them with educational materials. Pat says the airlines would often overlook their overweight luggage when she showed them that it was full of children's books and CDs.

Unfortunately, the resort where they'd stayed for so many years was closed when the US economy took a downward turn. Although they don't travel to Jamaica as often anymore, their trust fund for the Duncan School and "footprints" program to find shoes for every child lives on. By sharing her compassion with other members of their group, Pat and Bernie's vacation has resulted in thousands of kids getting a better education and a chance for a better life.

In 2005, Pat brought her compassion for children closer to home. Her son was attending an underperforming high school, so his chance of being accepted at a top college was not likely. With outside tutoring, her son improved and so did his potential of going to college.

Pat didn't stop at increasing her son's potential. She became active on the school board and worked to establish annual scholarships for high school sophomores and juniors

A DAILY DIFFERENCE

that would provide them with the tutoring that helped her son excel and get into college. In addition, Pat helped to establish scholarships for low-income graduating seniors who needed help paying for their books at the local community college.

Even though only one of her sons attended the high school and graduated in 2006, Pat still works with the school in an advisory position to ensure that the programs she started keep going with administrator and parent involvement. She still helps to fund the scholarships each year and has recruited others to help. The scholarships at the under-performing school have increased the number of seniors going to college by 22%.

Once you become active in helping others, you begin to think differently. Things that you've done for years can suddenly become ways to generate revenue for the cause you are supporting.

At a recent REO4Kids mastermind meeting, Pat volunteered to take responsibility for finding the conference room and discounted hotel rooms. It's common for hotels to give the conference organizer a free hotel room during the event, but Pat got them to include a free *suite*. Rather than take it herself, she found a creative way to turn the suite into a fundraiser for charity.

Pat decided to sell raffle tickets for the room to the 18 members participating in the mastermind event. She priced the tickets at $20 apiece and you could buy as many as you wanted. The winner received two prizes; the use of the suite

CHAPTER 11 – LEAVING FOOTPRINTS

for two days and the right to choose the children's charity that would benefit from the $360 collected in the raffle.

Every day there are opportunities like this to raise money for charity. Some require more creativity than others but if you continually look for ways to help others, you'll be surprised at what you can do. With a little thought and effort you can turn your time, talents, and tangible items into an unexpected gift for someone less fortunate.

How important is having a larger room for two days when the same money could be used to keep a kid off the street and out of gangs? That's what the money raised could buy at the Boys and Girls Clubs.

The next time something unexpected comes your way, find a way to share it with others or turn it into a charitable gift. The feeling you get from helping someone in need will last a lot longer than the distant memory of an oversized room. Pat has created footprints that will last long after she is gone. She has affected the lives of children in Jamaica, San Diego, and now Tucson.

12

Dream Maker

"The charitable give out the door and God puts it back through the window."– Source Unknown

A DAILY DIFFERENCE

Terry Rasner-Yacenda, in Reno, Nevada, is a dreamer. The only difference between Terry and the rest of the world is that she invests the time to conduct research, discovery, analysis, social trending, financing, legal structure, etc. to make her dreams come true.

Terry's inspiration and passion for giving comes from her mother, Christine, who always cared about and supported the underdogs, those down-and-out people who have been cast away even though they were in need of compassion. Terry's passion for helping others began as a volunteer for youth sports programs and expanded to include faith-based community outreach and feeding programs and in-hospital volunteering to assist in the social and emotional care of patients.

In 1997, Nevada Governor, Bob Miller, needed someone with the passion and heart to market a federal and state-funded health insurance program called "Nevada Check Up" to serve tens of thousands of uninsured children. He called on Terry to market the program to a population of skeptical public officials, health care providers, state legislators, the state's twenty-six Native American tribes, and low-income families with children in need of comprehensive medical, dental, vision, and counseling services.

Terry traveled the breadth and length of Nevada marketing Nevada Check Up, taking on the critics and naysayers, as thousands of children become enrolled. She often visited inner-city, high-risk neighborhoods to meet with community leaders, and brought along candy, toys, games,

CHAPTER 12 – DREAM MAKER

and her own money for the kids. She even used her own paper products to make signs and flyers announcing upcoming meetings and get-togethers. With overwhelming odds against her, Terry's efforts were successful. What started as a dream came to fruition and the Nevada Check Up program still exists today. For more information on Nevada Check Up, go to: **www.nevadacheckup.nv.gov.**

In Job 33:15, a dream is likened to *a vision of the night.* Terry says that every good thought or idea starts with a seed planted deep within one's soul. Then, at an "ah-ha moment," the seed sprouts and the dream is birthed. That's exactly what happened for Terry! When she opened her real estate brokerage she named it (what else?) "Dreams Realty." The name doesn't represent Terry's dream to own a real estate company; it reflects her dream of having the ability to help make many people's dreams come true.

Her brokerage has had a long history of committing to charities and faith-based groups that serve individuals, children, and families. But one day, an agent in their company received news that her son had died in his sleep in another country. The lady had just spoken to her son the previous day and he was scheduled to return home the following day.

Now, she was faced with the gut-wrenching reality of her loss. Her heart ached and she was confused about what she needed to do. Sitting in Terry's office with her heart broken, she had received little guidance on *how* to have her son's body returned home, only that it was going to cost thousands of dollars that she didn't have.

A DAILY DIFFERENCE

Terry had lost a son and could empathize with her loss. As she sat consoling the woman, Terry knew that she could do more and would do more. After some investigation and expense, Terry made arrangements to have the lady's son returned home for a beautiful funeral service with his mother in attendance.

Terry's tax accountant applauded her compassion, but informed her that her expenses were not eligible as a federal tax deduction. The idea of a Dreams Foundation was already in Terry's subconscious, but this event fueled the need to bring it to fruition. Their foundation could help people on a much larger scale if the resources expended were tax deductible for the donors, so she and her husband began working to obtain a Nevada Non-Profit Corporation and the Federal 501(c)(3) designation. It has been a bumpy ride, but Dreams Foundation, Inc. has passed two IRS approval stages and is expected to receive its 501(c)(3) tax deductible status in 2012.

Terry is not alone in her passion for giving. Her husband, John Yacenda, had directed several non-profit organizations in the past, which included doing a substantial amount of work representing Native American Tribes in the funding and development of their health care programs. John has served on the boards of several non-profit organizations and as the Executive Director of several non-profits in the health & human services field. He is currently a Governor-appointed member of Nevada's Juvenile Justice Commission.

Terry's daughter, Sarah Carmona, works with Terry in Dreams Realty and is also a giver. Continuing in the legacy set

CHAPTER 12 – DREAM MAKER

by her grandmother and mother, Sarah supports various charities and faith-based organizations. She is passionate about promoting diversity in the community by devoting time to serve on several boards and committees. Over the past two-and-a-half years, Dreams Realty has raised and donated $190,000 to benefit children and families.

Terry is known for her passionate approach to life and rarely turns away anyone who comes to her with a need. If she can't personally meet the need, she invests time in seeking another alternative to help the people through challenges that seem overwhelming to them. When I approached Terry about joining REO4Kids, ironically, she was on the same mission and was in the process of creating Dreams Foundation, Inc.

We expect that by combining the strengths and resources of REO4Kids with Dreams Foundation, Inc. a powerhouse of giving will result to improve the quality of life for many individuals, children, and families. It will be fun to watch us grow together. To find out more about Terry Rasner and Dreams Realty, go to: **www.dreamsrealty.net.**

13

Creating Hope

*"It is not what we get. But who we become,
what we contribute... that gives meaning to our lives."
– Anthony Robbins*

A DAILY DIFFERENCE

Steven Blackwood, in Little Rock, Arkansas, runs the top-selling real estate team in Arkansas. Steven attributes their business success to one thing - sharing with others. His most memorable childhood event occurred on Christmas when he was six years old. His family spent a good portion of their day filling green plastic garbage bags full of toys, clothing, bedding, and supplies to share with a family who had no running water in their home.

Steven's father was known by everyone in their community as a man with a passion for giving; who would give the "shirt off his back" to anyone in need. Steven says that somewhere along the line, his family's enthusiasm for giving went from being contagious to being "hereditary."

Steven and his wife, Cindi, have followed the family tradition by contributing to everything from "drug dog" training for their local police department, to building a bridge in a city park. They even donated a horse to fulfill a young child's Make-A-Wish request.

Since childhood, Steven had always found it easier to give than to receive. Although he was appreciative of the generosity of others, he struggled with being the recipient of their gifts. Several years ago, he began contacting people in advance of special occasions to request that in place of a gift, they make a contribution to a worthy cause.

He took the idea one step further in 1998 when, instead of spending the money on Christmas cards, he sent friends, clients, colleagues, affiliates, and family members a plain white

CHAPTER 13 – CREATING HOPE

envelope (the cheap kind that you can see through) with a ¼ sheet of 8½ " by 11"green paper that read:

"I have not purchased a Christmas card this year. In lieu of sending cards and gifts this Christmas, please know that a contribution has been made in your honor to provide Christmas for the children of a family in need. I do hope that you find my actions acceptable and I pray that you will have warmth and joy in knowing that some children will have a magical Christmas because of you."

Steven hoped to start a new trend or at least plant a seed that would inspire others to do the same. Not only was his idea well received, it prompted an array of phone calls, thank you notes and personal visits from those who felt compelled to thank him in person. A close friend has copied it every year since.

I was with Steven at a conference in Florida in October, 2008, when his world was turned upside down. He received the call that all parents dread; his son, Alex was dead, a victim of suicide. Steven hit his knees and was physically unable to function. Members of our REO4Kids group packed his bag and transported him to the airport for his dreadfully long flight home. Only those who have lost a child under these circumstances can understand the array of emotions that parents must go through.

I didn't see Steven again for more than a year and he was still visibly shaken. However, as time passed and the scars began to heal, Steven's passion for giving not only returned, it grew exponentially! If anything, their son's suicide has given

A DAILY DIFFERENCE

Steven more passion than he's ever had in his life. A photo of Alex is provided in Figure 13-1.

Figure 13-1 Alex Blackwood

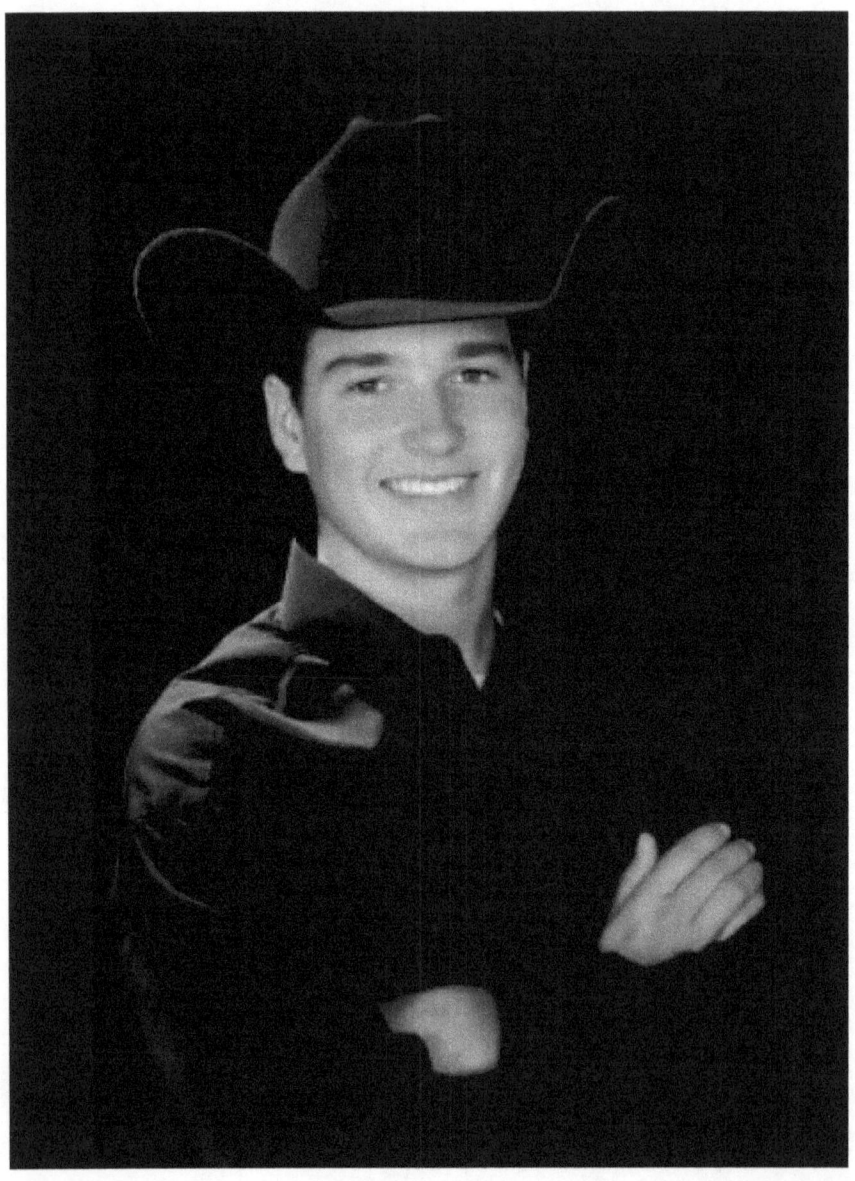

CHAPTER 13 – CREATING HOPE

At the urging of Alex's friends, Steven and Cindi created the Alex Blackwood Memorial Foundation for HOPE. Steven now spends about half of his time working to promote depression awareness and suicide prevention in hopes of keeping other families from experiencing the pain that he and his family had to endure.

Throughout this book I've paraphrased the comments of the friends I wrote about. I struggled with how to do that with Cindi Blackwood's comments and found that I couldn't do a better job than she had done in capturing her feelings. The *italicized* text below about losing her son and life in the aftermath was written by Cindi Blackwood:

Charitable contributions - The formality of those words is about exciting as they look on tax documents. But words such as sharing, giving, helping, investing in the lives of others... now those words sound much more meaningful.

Most of my life I have been involved in various church and community activities and organizations that have allowed me to participate in giving of my time and resources. But only in the last 3 1/2 years have these and more opportunities become much more meaningful to me. In October, 2008, our family experienced the greatest tragedy of our lives when we lost our 19 year-old son, Alex, to suicide. He was a charming, good-looking, bright young man with a world of potential at his disposal. To say we were shocked is an enormous understatement.

Even though my husband of 26+ years, Steven, has been much more involved in the Alex Blackwood Foundation, my awareness of the significance of being a part of charitable organizations has been tremendously expanded. And most importantly, my outlook on my own time and money invested has completely changed for the good. Now instead of viewing it as just a good deed, I truly appreciate the opportunity to give, share, and invest in the lives of others.

Recently I spoke at a Boys and Girls Club on behalf of the Alex Blackwood Foundation for Hope. That same week an article in the newspaper talked about students from the Boys and Girls Club who had received national recognition for their accomplishments in college, which they attributed to the club. As I reflected on the students in attendance when I spoke, I wondered which of them would go on to do great things in the world. Being able to be even a very small part of a child's success makes it all worthwhile.

In the beginning of the 2010/2011 school year, I began participating in an Encourager program which is a part of Step Ministries. Every Wednesday I go to a local elementary school and help two students assigned to me with math, reading or any other subject needing improvement. Before I began being an Encourager, I struggled with thoughts such as "Do I really have time for this? I'm so busy with work." After my first week, all of those thoughts changed and I look forward to the one hour each week that I get to spend with these students.

I always ask my students to tell me something good that has happened to them since the last time I saw them, or something fun they have done, or a way that they helped someone else. In the beginning they would say they didn't know of anything, but when I started to ask more questions, they quickly came up with something to tell me. Now, as soon as they see me they are smiling and cannot

CHAPTER 13 – CREATING HOPE

wait to tell me something good! That warms my heart and makes it all worthwhile! Being able to invest in the lives of these students is a privilege and I am honored to be a part of it.

Another group that I am still in the process of organizing is Moms with a Common Bond. After the loss of my son, I found comfort in seeking advice and encouragement from other mothers who have lost children. So many of the things I have struggled with seem crazy to other people who have not lost a child. We have just begun meeting and have already learned so much from each other and always leave encouraged. I have no idea what lies in store for this group but I know we all share the idea that helping others helps us!

What I've learned the most about giving to others whether it is time, money, or both, is that I am the one who benefits the most! I can't wait to tell my family and co-workers about "my kids" at McDermott Elementary and I proudly display their pictures in my office. If I am having a not-so-good day, once I see them, my whole perspective changes. Whenever I see a lemonade stand in a front yard or a bake sale raising money for kids to go to a camp or a sports tournament, or a Salvation Army bell ringer at Christmas, I can't wait to help, even if it's just giving the change in my purse. I believe we are put on this earth to help others. The joy we receive is a bonus... a very big bonus!!!

Prior to losing Alex, Steven had always given his gifts anonymously to ensure that the recipients wouldn't try to pay him back. After Alex died, he realized that good ideas for helping people need to be shared. Steven believes that most people want to help others, but don't know how. They need

A DAILY DIFFERENCE

someone to set an example that paves the way for others to follow. The answer is always going to be "no" if you never ask!

Steven's advice is not to let the fear of "what if," prevent you from taking action. If you have an idea or an opportunity to help someone, do it! Your fear of what people might think robs the recipient of a gift and you of the joy of giving it. A gift ungiven, actions not taken, friendly smiles or gestures unshared, or kind words unspoken are wasted opportunities to make someone's day brighter. Here are Steven's seven ways to make the world a better place.

1) Pay it forward - don't let fear stop you
2) Commit a random act of kindness today - every day
3) Never underestimate the power of encouragement
4) Be sensitive to those around you
5) Look for opportunities to do little things for people
6) Dare to be different
7) Be the change you wish to see in this world

Instead of allowing themselves to become victims of their tragedy, Steven and Cindi Blackwood have embraced it to honor the all-too-short life of their 19 year-old son, Alex. They funded a statewide on-line emotional support system to help diagnose depression and treat it before it progresses to suicide. The "Connect Without Cost" program ensures that "at risk" teens (and adults) are seen by a counselor or therapist without concern for the cost of the initial assessment. When a financial hardship exists, they seek donors and help to arrange scholarships to cover the cost of follow-up care.

CHAPTER 13 – CREATING HOPE

Steven has become a national spokesperson for suicide prevention. His passionate mission to overcome the stigma of depression is "breaking the silence" and saving lives. Steven has appeared on local television news and was interviewed by Anderson Cooper on CNN. In 2011, he received a national award for his grassroots efforts from the American Foundation for Suicide Prevention. To keep up with the efforts of Steven and Cindi Blackwood go to: **www.theblackwoodteam.com**.

Steven and Cindi have supported every charity fundraiser I've held and Camille and I have supported the Alex Blackwood Foundation's "Ride for Hope" fundraiser every year since inception. I suspect that we're sending the same money back and forth every year but it's nice to have people who you can always count on.

If there's a lesson to be learned with the Blackwoods, it's that life isn't about what happens to you; it's about how you *deal* with what happens to you. I can't tell you how much I respect and admire Steven and Cindi Blackwood for turning their terrible loss into an opportunity to help others. For more information about the Alex Blackwood Foundation for Hope go to: **www.alexblackwoodfoundation.org**.

14

The Gift of Compassion

"It is possible to give without loving, but it is impossible to love without giving." – Richard Braunsteing

A DAILY DIFFERENCE

I met Lauren Border at a real estate conference in Dallas, Texas, in 2010. She was the coordinator for the conference where we were exhibiting and came by our booth several times over the three-day event to ensure that everything was going well. Lauren acted in a professional manner, but I could tell by her enthusiasm that she was genuinely passionate about helping people. We became friends and as I've gotten to know her, I have realized that she is an amazing human being.

Lauren knows first-hand what it feels like to receive help from others. As the child of struggling young parents, every day was a challenge for her family. Charity was certainly no stranger to their household; it wasn't then and it isn't now.

Help came from many places, including government assistance with food stamps, reduced-price lunches at school, and neighbors dropping by unexpectedly with extra food and clothing. Lauren grew up with a sincere appreciation of the society that had constantly assisted her family.

Suffering in childhood is not a prerequisite to giving as an adult, but I've found that many who have been helped by others seem to be on a lifelong mission to return the favor. The great thing about helping others is that it provides the same warm feeling of accomplishment regardless of where you come from. Lauren learned to accept help and to help others whenever she could.

While in college at the University of Oklahoma, Lauren and others in her sorority participated in a philanthropy project sponsored by the National Education Association called

CHAPTER 14 – THE GIFT OF COMPASSION

"Read Across America." The program promotes children's literacy by reading with children, holding various fundraisers, and conducting book drives to ensure that kids will have enough materials to read. For more information on Read Across America, go to **www.readacrossamerica.org**.

Many people have the misconception that charitable giving means opening your checkbook. Lauren learned that you can be just as effective by setting aside a few hours each month to help someone who needs it. Giving your time, especially to children, is just as important, probably more important, than making a monetary contribution.

Lauren paid her own way through college with the help of student loans and graduated in 2008 with a degree in Journalism. Even though she's had a job for several years, she uses a substantial portion of her income to pay back the Sallie Mae loans each month. While she's made it a priority to pay off her college debt, she did not let her financial limitations get in the way of helping others.

Upon graduating from college, Lauren began volunteering with the Big Brothers Big Sisters program. She was matched with an amazing little girl named Ebony. During their first year together, Lauren and Ebony typically met three or four times a month, and over time developed a fabulous relationship. Whether going to a bookstore, doing homework together, eating, or just talking, Lauren says that spending time with Ebony has been one of the greatest blessings in her life. There is something to be said about seeing life through the eyes of a 7-year old.

A DAILY DIFFERENCE

During their second year together in Big Brothers Big Sisters, Lauren volunteered to coach a recreational cheer squad so Ebony could join the team free of charge. Being on a competitive squad taught Ebony many valuable lessons. She also received free gymnastics lessons from Lauren's stepfather, Victor, and together, they've experienced many great things. The only cost to build a lifetime of memories was Lauren's investment of time. She'll be the first to tell you that she received far more than she gave!

The Big Brothers Big Sisters program helps their sponsoring adults, referred to as "Bigs," by enrolling them in a discount program which provides access to a multitude of arts and crafts, local events, restaurants, etc. The organization goes out of their way to support the adults who support their kids. They are constantly sending emails with information about many free activities. For more information about Big Brothers Big Sisters go to: **www.bbbs.org.**

Ebony will soon be 10 years old and already has dreams of going to college. She was recently elected to the Student Council and the National Elementary Honor Society. Lauren's investment of time has made a positive impact on Ebony. She is no longer the shy 7-year old that Lauren first met three years ago. Ebony has blossomed into a talkative, honor student with a heart of gold.

Lauren stops short of taking credit for these achievements because Ebony has an amazing mother who does everything she can for her daughter, even though she's a single mom. Lauren gets excited just talking about Ebony and her

CHAPTER 14 – THE GIFT OF COMPASSION

mother and is thankful that they've been such a blessing in her life. It's amazing to consider the impact just a few hours a month can have on people. A photo of Ebony and Lauren is provided in Figure 14-1.

Figure 14-1 Lauren Border and Ebony

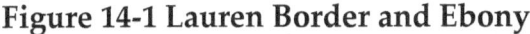

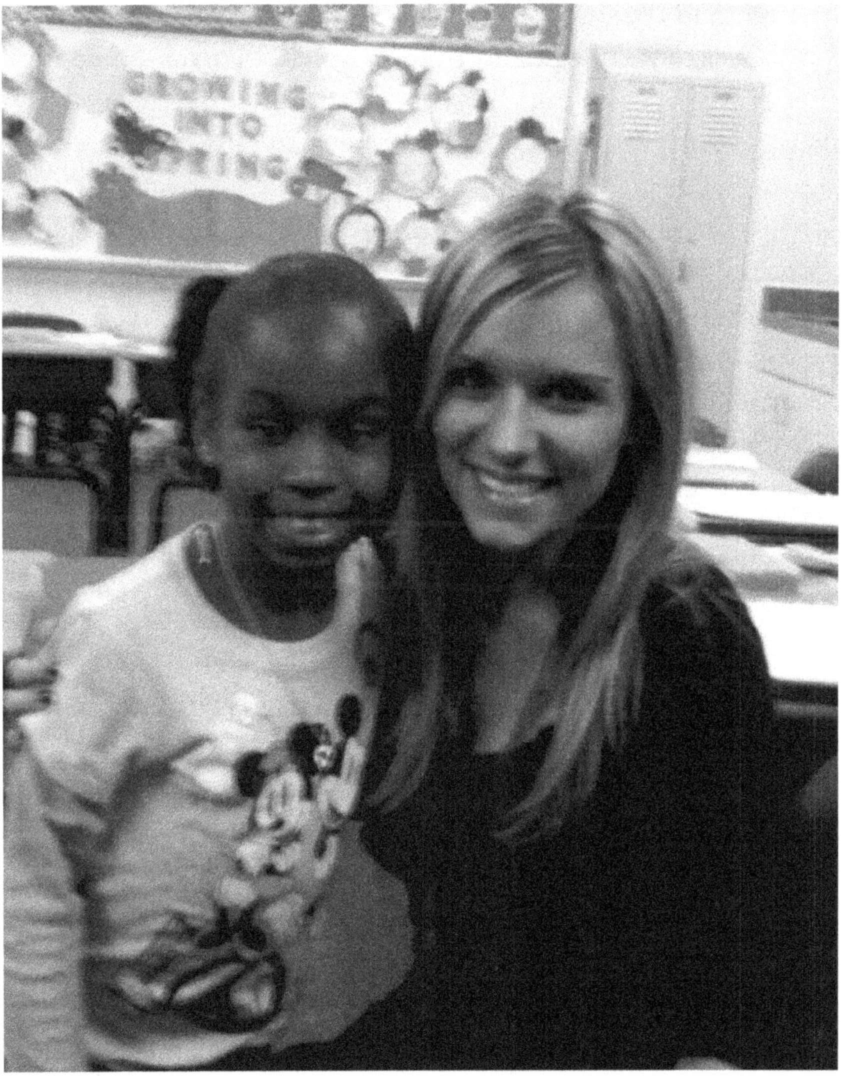

A DAILY DIFFERENCE

The people who helped Lauren's family when she was growing up did more than just feed them; they helped an entire family achieve success! Lauren's step-father, Victor, worked two jobs while attending college. Without the help his family received, he would have had to drop out of college to get a third job in order to provide enough food for Lauren, her mother, and two brothers. Instead, her step-father was able to graduate from college and become a school teacher. He now shapes the lives of middle school children and teaches them the discipline required to participate in gymnastics.

Lauren's mother, Andrea, went to college while working full-time and went on to become the Vice President of Operations at a telecommunications company. Lauren graduated from college and is the National Account Executive for Housing Wire magazine. Her brother, Bryson, graduated from college recently and her youngest brother, Alexander, is a college athlete who will graduate in 2013.

Who knows what would have happened to this young family had they not been surrounded by compassionate people in a society that nurtures those who need it. You'll never know in advance whether your kindness will make a difference for a day or completely alter a family's destiny.

Those who helped Lauren's family will continue to make a difference for centuries as their gift of compassion is passed on to other families, future generations, and a shy 7-year old named Ebony. Kindness and the hard work of Lauren's parents took this family from low-skill jobs to leadership positions in companies and their community.

15

A Dollar A Day

"He who waits to do a great deal of good at once, will never do anything." – Samuel Johnson

A DAILY DIFFERENCE

I spent several years teaching personal finance to 6th and 7th grade children through the Junior Achievement Program. I targeted 12 and 13 year-olds because they were just starting to earn their own money by doing odd jobs like babysitting, lawn maintenance, newspaper delivery, etc. I hoped to teach them about saving and making charitable donations before they learned to spend all that they earned, as soon as they earned it.

I challenged each student in my class to save one dollar a day, but many didn't think that they could do it. To show them how easy it could be, I asked them how much it would cost to buy a 20 oz. soft drink from the dispensing machines in the hallway, and then how much it cost to get a drink from the water fountain. The answer was obvious.

Next, I asked how many of them ordered a glass of water when they went out to eat with their parents. Very few said that they did, so as a homework assignment, I asked them to find out whether their parents would be willing to put $1.00 in their savings account every time they ordered water at a restaurant rather than a soft drink.

The results were not surprising; all of the parents said that they would invest the money for their child. Wouldn't it be better for the money to be in your child's savings account or helping a charitable institution rather than in the restaurant owner's cash register? Water is better for you anyway; it doesn't rot your teeth or lead to obesity.

CHAPTER 15 – A DOLLAR A DAY

Let's calculate how much this one simple change could add to your annual budget. If a family of four ate at a restaurant twice a month, and the cost of a soda, coffee, or other beverage was $1.00 per serving, a savings of $4.00 would result from each visit. Eating out every other week is 26 meals per year, so the savings would be $104.00 ($4.00 x 26 visits = $104.00), but that isn't all!

You will probably pay sales tax on your purchase of about 8%. You would also give your server a tip; probably 15%. With added expenses of 23%, the real cost of your family's drinks is $127.92 per year ($104 x 23% = $23.92 + $104.00 = $127.92).

Once the students were convinced that they could find creative ways to save, I challenged them to find a way to save a dollar every day for three years. Between employment income, birthday cash, and revenue from their parents for ordering water, it would not be that difficult. I told them to plan for a month off from saving in December, to purchase Christmas gifts for their family.

If they could save a dollar a day for 334 days of the year, they'd have $334 at the end of the year (365 days per year – 31 days in December = 334 days of saving). If they could accomplish this for three years, their savings account would total $1,000 (plus interest). For more information about Junior Achievement, go to **www.ja.org**.

Most people know that they should be saving for the future and giving to charitable causes but life gets in the way.

A DAILY DIFFERENCE

When teens get out of high school, many go to college. When they finish college and find a job, they buy a new car and new furniture. This puts them into debt immediately, which requires monthly interest and principle payments.

Because they aren't studying every night, they develop a social calendar which involves eating out, going to sporting events, concerts, and other night life activities. They also take up hobbies and begin to acquire music, movies, books, clothing, etc., all of which require money.

When they fall in love, they'll spend money on travel, gifts, and outings together. The next logical step is a wedding, and that usually means finding a bigger place to live. The additional square footage requires more furniture, draperies, appliances, and décor, as well as more utility usage, and higher insurance. Once settled, they start families and have new expenses for daycare, diapers, healthcare, etc. Each pay raise is quickly used to pay for sporting equipment, karate lessons, doll houses, or gymnastics training.

After eighteen years of never-ending bills, their children finally turn 18 years-old and finish high school, but many parents feel obligated to help them with college expenses so they can get a job and move out! During college or after graduation, they'll meet their soul mates, fall in love, and have wedding expenses; which parents also feel obligated to pay.

When their children are finally educated, have a good job, and a home of their own, the parents take a big sigh of relief... before the grandchildren come!

CHAPTER 15 – A DOLLAR A DAY

It's very easy to get caught up in living and forget to save or help others. You'd be surprised how many people don't start planning their retirement until they turn 55 years old! Many *never* make the time for planned giving.

In 2010, I was interviewed by a local television station at a Boys & Girls Club facility in Tucson, Arizona. The entire facility, complete with gymnasium, computer lab, classrooms, and equipment had been donated, yet they had to cancel sports leagues and close the facility a few days each month because of budget cuts. I asked the reporter, "Don't you think it's pathetic that this magnificent gift is being wasted because our city of *one million people* can't donate enough money to pay the staff?"

If each Tucson resident would give just one dollar per month, we could raise $12 million dollars annually and build several new Clubhouses each year to keep at-risk kids in school, off the streets, and out of gangs. That's the trouble with society - everyone expects that *someone else* will give.

Charitable efforts need be a planned part of your monthly budget. It is very difficult for non-profit organizations to create a budget, lease facilities, and hire staff to accomplish their mission if they don't know how much money they will have to spend.

Most charitable organizations rely on checks of $25 or less to keep their doors open. Because their income is unpredictable, they must constantly work to get people to see them on television (which costs money), hear them on the

A DAILY DIFFERENCE

radio (which costs money) or realize their accomplishments through mailings (which cost money).

No amount is too small, as long as it is *consistent!* When charities have consistent donations, they can spend fewer resources on advertising and more on accomplishing their mission and developing revenue streams that add stability.

The people featured throughout this book were able to raise substantial amounts of money, but nearly all of it came over time from small donations. It's not big checks that make a difference; it's the *consistent* checks. Do what you can; but do *something*.

The quote on the first page of this chapter by Samuel Johnson is worth repeating, "He who waits to do a great deal of good at once, will never do anything."

16

Small Change, Big Difference

"The Dead Sea is the dead sea, because it continually receives and never gives." - Source Unknown

A DAILY DIFFERENCE

When you make a commitment to help others, it helps to create a plan for giving. Ramsey Fahel (Chapter 1) saved his loose change in advance because he planned to the drop the coins where others would find them. He *planned* to make a difference that day.

The first thing to decide is how you will make a difference and then plan your actions. When Mike and Kathy Bell, parents of Lizzie Bell (Chapter 5), were in Chicago for their daughter's wedding in 2011, they packed $25 in small bills and coins so they would be able to help the homeless people on the street as they moved through the city - 25 cents here, a dollar there.

When the money was gone it was gone; but they planned to make the difference and then acted. No one knew they were doing this but they knew - because it was a priority for them. They're able to do things like this regularly because giving is important to them and they plan for it in their budget.

When I was volunteering for Junior Achievement, my favorite part of the curriculum was the class on budgeting. For this class, I'd divide the 6th and 7th graders into five "families" and then have each family choose a folded slip of paper from my hand. The slips of paper indicated the level of education each family's wage earner had achieved: High School diploma, Associate of Science degree, Bachelor of Science degree, Masters degree, or Doctorate degree.

The family with the high school education was given a budget of $1,000 per month. The family with the two-year

CHAPTER 16 – SMALL CHANGE, BIG DIFFERENCE

degree received $2,000 per month. The four-year degreed family earned $3,000 per month, the family with the graduate degree earned $4,000, and the family with the PhD earned $5,000 per month. This exercise was an excellent way for the kids to understand the economic difference higher education can make.

The family with a high school education would usually become quite vocal about the perceived unfairness in income distribution, so I'd have to explain to them that employers pay more for knowledge; the more knowledge you have, the more valuable you are in the job market. Whoever coined the phrase "Knowledge is Power" was right when it comes to wages.

Each family would be tasked with making their income match their expenditures in the following categories: Housing, Taxes, Transportation, Food, Clothing, Healthcare, Savings, Charity, and Family Discretion. I projected a pie chart provided by the Junior Achievement organization on the overhead screen that showed the amount spent on each expense category, based on national averages at the time.

At the end of the class, I'd ask a representative of each family to report on how they'd allocated their money. Every time I taught this class, the High School-educated family, with an income of only $1,000, would come to the conclusion that they couldn't afford a car. They would opt to save the money they'd otherwise spend on car payments, license plates, collision insurance, gasoline, and depreciation by riding the bus. The money they saved allowed them to spend more for housing, which resulted in a larger home in a nicer area.

A DAILY DIFFERENCE

This was the first realization for many of the kids that so little of what they earned would be available for them to spend after all the bills were paid. I think this exercise made them appreciate their parents a little more and helped them to understand why their parents couldn't always provide them with everything that they asked for.

The lesson in this exercise is that life is about choices. You have only a limited amount of time and money to spend. When you choose to spend time or money in one place, you lose the ability to spend it anywhere else. This is commonly referred to as an "opportunity cost."

Most people know exactly where their income comes from (their job) but don't have a clear idea of where it all goes, so they don't know until it's too late that one expenditure will cost them the ability to make another. If they used a budget, they'd know, but mentioning the word "budget" to most people makes them *cringe*. They immediately think, "Spend less" but this isn't always true.

Having a budget will allow you to spend <u>more</u> on the things you enjoy like vacations, vehicles, hobbies, and charitable contributions because it allows you to *plan* for them rather than hope that there is money left for them after other bills are paid.

A budget is simply a tool to balance your earnings with your expenditures. Having a clear understanding of your finances allows you to spend more, if you spend wisely. By

CHAPTER 16 – SMALL CHANGE, BIG DIFFERENCE

eliminating wasteful spending you could have the money to do the things you like and be financially able to help others.

How much could be saved by making sandwiches at home rather than eating lunch in a restaurant? If your charitable plan was to feed the homeless, you could use some of the savings from making your own sandwiches to make extra sandwiches every day and give them to homeless people on the street who have no food. You could *save money* while helping someone! Charitable acts don't have to cost money.

The average American watches 20 hours of television each week, which is equal to 50% of the time spent working at a full time job! If you think you don't have time to help others, just think how productive you could become if you spent 20 hours each week helping people instead of staring into a box that gives you unexplainable cravings for junk food, jewelry, and music from 30 years ago! The true cost of television isn't the monthly bill; it's the lost opportunity to do something productive with your time.

17

Passionate Planning

"As the purse is emptied, the heart is filled." – Victor Hugo

A DAILY DIFFERENCE

Hopefully your creative juices are flowing, and you're thinking of how you can help people. There are endless opportunities, but it's important to find a cause that you're passionate about. Think of an injustice, disease, disaster, or other situation that really bothers you; something you would work on for years to resolve. Whatever you are most passionate about should become your mission. Camille and I made a decision to focus our efforts on improving the lives of children because kids are *born* with or into their problems. If someone doesn't do something to change their outcome, the problem could be passed along for generations.

In order to achieve consistent success, goals must be established, written, and tracked. You wouldn't load your family into your car and start driving on a long trip without having a destination (or at least a direction) in mind. You should have a map of how to reach your destination and a vague idea of the progress you intend to make each day. *Hope* is <u>not</u> a business plan! You need to have a written plan of what you wish to accomplish so your can track your progress.

The goals you set can be the difference between success and failure! Aiming too low with an easily achievable goal isn't challenging so it's easy to become bored and lose interest. Setting a goal that is too high can cause you to become discouraged if you fail to achieve it. A good goal should be difficult but achievable, spread over time, and broken into the smallest measurable pieces possible. All goals, whether small or large should be in line with your long-term goal.

CHAPTER 17 – PASSIONATE PLANNING

Goals should be SMART (Specific, Measurable, Achievable, Realistic, and Time-bound). If someone says, "I want to lose weight," this is certainly an excellent goal, but it's far too vague. Keep the SMART acronym in mind when setting your goals. Get started by determining what you want to accomplish and when you want to have it done. What are your long-term objectives? These are things you want to accomplish in a year.

Once you've set the long-term goal, establish short-term goals; monthly, weekly and daily actions that will move you toward the long-term objectives. Be careful not to push too hard or too fast and set yourself up for failure. Your goals are your road map. Follow them and you'll be well on your way!

After your goals are established, they need to be communicated to others who can help you achieve them. The United Way does a great job of communicating their fundraising progress with their visual "thermometer" charts. The red in the bulb of the thermometer steadily creeps up the long slender tube as more and more donations are received. The charts are posted in a variety of locations to give the community an update of how well they are doing at reaching their goal.

If you tell the average person that you're trying to raise $100,000, you might as well say that the goal is $100 million because most people can't relate well to either number. The first thing to do is break the goal into *fifty weeks*. I know that a year has 52 weeks, but most people encounter more expenses around Christmas. By accomplishing their giving over the first

A DAILY DIFFERENCE

fifty weeks of the year, they can use the money they would normally donate to pay for the increased travel, shopping, and food expenditures most families face at the end of the year.

Splitting the $100,000 goal into fifty weeks reduces it to $2,000 per week. Spreading the $2,000 weekly goal over five work days reduces the amount to $400 per work day, which is a more manageable number. If 20 people who are committed to the goal would pledge to lead a small fundraising team, the daily goal would be reduced to $20 per team. If each team leader got 10 of their friends, co-workers, and family members to pledge $2 per work day the goal would be achieved.

Giving $2 per day is easier than you might think, especially when you consider that your donation is probably deductible on your income tax. If you're in a 25% tax bracket, you really only have to save $1.50 per day because the other 50 cents comes back in an income tax refund that you wouldn't have gotten otherwise.

Having a regular coffee every other day instead of one topped with whipped cream and caramel would save more than enough to make up the difference. As illustrated in Chapter 15, having a glass of water at meals instead of an unhealthy soft drink is another way to raise the money.

When you consider the difference you can make in someone's life by simply foregoing an unhealthy beverage each day, it makes you feel kind of guilty for having it the first place, especially if your donation is being matched by the other people on your team and the 190 people on the other teams.

CHAPTER 17 – PASSIONATE PLANNING

Let's say that we had a goal to grant 52 wishes this year for the Make-A-Wish Foundation® and the average cost of each wish is $7,000. This is how I would organize the "Wish-A-Week" campaign:

52 weeks X $7,000/wish = $364,000 total needed
1) Get 52 individuals or groups to become "Wand Wavers" (wish granters) who take responsibility for raising $7,000 in the next 12 months to grant one wish. (This is not as hard as it sounds - 27 people pledging $5 per week = $7,000. Use a slogan like, "Change from LUNCH can change a LIFE!")

2) Get local companies to do a "Wish Match" to match the funds raised by the Wand Waver teams (Each company pledges a percentage match of each wish funded. If a company pledges a 1% match, they pay $70 for every wish the Wand Wavers fund). Some companies may commit to match 3%, 5%, or even 10% because they are *matching* work done by others, not being asked to do it all themselves! For every wish funded by the Wand Wavers, another is matched, so TWO wishes are granted! For every fifty cents either group gives, a dollar is raised.

3) Create press releases every month and every time you reach a major $100K milestone. Use the media to acknowledge the efforts of the Wand Wavers and Wish Match companies. Positive reinforcement causes everyone to work harder. Positive press for companies reduces their need to advertise, so they can give even more!

18

Get Optimistic!

"Whether you think you can or think you can't, either way you are right."– Henry Ford

A DAILY DIFFERENCE

I became a member of the Optimist Club by accident. I'd shared Gena Foster's flocking story (Chapter 2) with my friends, Joel Trupiano and Amanda Smicklas, and they invited me to share the story with the members of their local Optimist Club. After visiting the club and sharing Gena's story, Camille and I learned about all the good things the Optimist Club is doing for local kids. We joined Optimist International because it seemed like their goal of helping children aligned well with ours.

Several of the Optimist Club members were so excited about bringing the flamingos to Tucson that we used some of my book proceeds to buy 100 flamingos, which could make 4 "flocks" of 25 birds each. I intend to use the flamingos to assist local high school teams, charities, scouts, etc. in their fundraising efforts.

Non-profit groups wanting to raise money will check the birds out free-of-charge. The kids doing the flocking will keep *half* the proceeds they raise. The other half of the money will go to the Optimist Club to fund other youth-related activities. At 50%, the split for the non-profit is much better than they typically receive by selling cookie dough (Chapter 3), coupon books, popcorn, or other items, and the kids who are granted free use of the flamingos are "paying it forward" to other kids being funded by the Optimist Club.

Each supporter of your charitable group should go to the businesses they frequently visit to ask for a matching gift. You should start by briefly explaining the issue the charity is trying to address. Next, let them know that you have the

CHAPTER 18 – GET OPTIMISTIC!

solution but need their help to make the solution a reality. The script would sound something like this. *"It costs the Boys and Girls Club $500 per year for each child we take off the street and into our clubhouses. These kids are taught to be responsible, sharing human beings. For every $500 we raise in grass roots efforts, can I count on you for a 5% match? That's only $25 for every $500 we raise to keep a child in school and out of gangs."* If you were able to get 20 businesses to pay 5%, you would DOUBLE the money the kids raised putting up the flamingos!

If the kids compiled the name and address of all the homeowners who paid them to move the flamingos, a letter could be sent thanking them for their support. The letter would also include a list of the 20 businesses that matched the homeowner's donation and politely ask that they frequent these businesses to ensure that they can continue to support the community. If you recruited 20 additional businesses for matching gifts on the second year, the match would be 200% of what the kids raise!

People love bargains. On the days after major holidays, they line up for hours, even days, to get discounts of 30, 40, or 50%. When every dollar they give is *tripled*, it's like finding a 66% off sale! Since everyone's gift is being tripled, people will probably donate more.

It's a lot easier to raise money with a group than it is by yourself. A great place to meet and network with other positive, sharing people who want to make a difference is at your local Optimist Club. I was pleased and surprised to find that each meeting is started by standing and reciting the

A DAILY DIFFERENCE

Pledge of Allegiance. Sometime during the past few decades, kids stopped reciting the "Pledge" in schools like I did every day from first grade through high school. It's refreshing to find a group willing to acknowledge their allegiance to the flag that represents the freedoms we enjoy that allow us to prosper.

Optimist Club meetings are short, productive, and inspiring. The meetings serve as planning sessions for local fundraising efforts and updates on state, regional, and national campaigns. I highly recommend finding a club in your area. Your involvement will improve your outlook on life and positively impact the lives of others in your community. I leave each meeting feeling better about myself for being more aware of the challenges faced by those around me.

At the end of each meeting, members stand and recite the Optimist's Creed, which is provided below:

OPTIMIST CREED
Promise Yourself...

To be so strong that nothing can disturb your peace of mind.

To talk health, happiness and prosperity to every person you meet.

To make all your friends feel that there is something in them.

To look at the sunny side of everything and make your optimism come true.

To think only of the best, to work only for the best, and to expect only the best.

CHAPTER 18 – GET OPTIMISTIC!

To be just as enthusiastic about the success of others as you are about your own.

To forget the mistakes of the past and press on to the greater achievements of the future.

To wear a cheerful countenance at all times and give every living creature you meet a smile.

To give so much time to the improvement of yourself that you have no time to criticize others.

To be too large for worry, too noble for anger, too strong for fear, and too happy to permit the presence of trouble.

19

Challenge Yourself!

"I hope that my achievements in life shall be these - that I will have fought for what was right and fair, that I will have risked for that which mattered, and that I will have given help to those who were in need, that I will have left the earth a better place for what I've done and who I've been." – C. Hoppe

A DAILY DIFFERENCE

I've heard the expression, *"birds of a feather flock together"* since I was a child, but never really knew what it meant until I started sharing. Through helping others, I have met some very generous people who were willing to share.

Sure, several people took what I'd shared without reciprocating, but that is expected. All seeds don't find fertile ground. Those who respond to kindness with kindness of their own will single themselves out as the people with whom you want to become friends.

Surrounding yourself with a network of like-minded people will build a support group that can be instrumental in helping you achieve your goals. When the people in your group take action, it will inspire you to drum up the courage to follow their example.

Whenever I've taken on a challenging task, I tell everyone I know what I plan to do. Public proclamations are responsible for helping me achieve some of my toughest goals. After telling everyone that I would write this book in a *month*, I finished writing it in a week and had it <u>published</u> in a month! Holding yourself accountable works!

When you make a public proclamation, pay attention to how the people around you respond. This is a good way of determining who your friends really are. Those who are small-minded or jealous of your accomplishments may be afraid that you're going to pass them in status. They won't be supportive of your goals and will privately hope that you fail. Because

CHAPTER 19 – CHALLENGE YOURSELF!

these people have never had the courage to change their own situation, your success will make them feel like a failure.

Don't let these people get you down. Surround yourself with genuine friends who have a positive attitude and are supportive of your ambitions. True friends will help you to succeed at your endeavors and tell you when you're making a mistake. Their encouragement will lift your spirits and increase your commitment to follow through and complete what you set out to do.

When recruiting other people to join you, the message should never be conveyed as, "look what I did," but rather, "look what YOU can do!" You have to lead in order for people to follow, and there is no bigger motivator than a previous track record of results.

In order to achieve that track record, you *must* make mistakes. There's a big difference between theory and practice. Not much can be learned from someone who has never done what you want to accomplish. I'd much rather be *shown* what has worked than instructed about what *should* work.

You'll *never* give to a charitable group if you don't believe that you can afford it, so keep an open mind to possibilities. Improving the lives of children has been my motivation for sharing our fundraising successes and failures in this book. I hope that reading about some of the simple things others have done will inspire you to do something, too!

A DAILY DIFFERENCE

In Chapter 1, Ramsey Fahel dropped loose change on the ground to provide a smile in other people's day and John Fox showed people how to bring out the best in themselves.

In Chapter 2, Gena Foster raised money with her son, one flamingo at a time, to help cancer victims.

In Chapter 3, Ron Gamble inspired a congregation to give by offering skills and materials to rewire a church camp.

In Chapter 4, Joann Bersell, Debbie Turner, and their team donated their time to raise money at a charity auction.

In Chapter 5, Lizzie Bell and Camden Garcia turned their Make-A-Wish® experience into a crusade to help others.

In Chapter 6, REO4Kids members combined their efforts to change the lives of thousands of kids, one house at a time.

In Chapter 7, Amy Coleman & Bruce Hammer collected $4,500 in loose change and checks for charity just by asking.

In Chapter 8, Lester and Patricia Cox helped to keep a faltering Big Sisters chapter alive by refusing to quit.

In Chapter 9, Teresa Ryan led by example to inspire a community to donate $2 million dollars in hurricane relief.

In Chapter 10, Nancy Braun transformed a training class she was required to teach into a fundraising activity.

In Chapter 11, Pat Koch turned a vacation into a crusade to buy shoes and educational materials for destitute children.

In Chapter 12, Terry Rasner-Yacenda created Dreams Foundation, Inc. to help people who fall through the cracks.

In Chapter 13, Steven and Cindi Blackwood turned their personal tragedy it into an opportunity to create awareness.

In Chapter 14, Lauren Border and her family returned the goodness shown to them by making an impact on others.

In Chapter 15, grade school kids learned how saving a dollar a day can provide a consistent donation to a charity.

CHAPTER 19 – CHALLENGE YOURSELF!

None of these efforts required "rocket science," - just a strong desire to make a difference, a plan to divide the task into small achievable pieces, and the commitment to make it happen. You can do it, too! All you need to do is ACT: create **A**wareness, have **C**ompassion, and **T**ake action! The simple three-step formula is provided below:

    Awareness
    Compassion
    Take Action

    Better World

I'd like to challenge you to **make the time to make a difference** in someone's life. It will reward you beyond belief.

If you've enjoyed reading this book, please share it with others and get the word out by leaving a positive review at: **www.amazon.com/Bob-Zachmeier/e/B0044P1FIY**.

If you would like to use this book in your fundraising efforts, send an e-mail to **bob@bobzachmeier.com**. I will sell this book to charitable groups for cost (approximately 80% off the cover price). Your charitable group can keep anything over the cost of printing and shipping the books!

Pay It Forward!

Bob Zachmeier

INDEX
People and Entities

Name	Page
Alex Blackwood	97,99-102
Alex Blackwood Foundation for HOPE	98
Amanda Smiklas	x,128
American Foundation for Suicide Prevention	102
Amy Coleman	ix,40,41,52-54,56,58,59,64,136
Anthony Robbins	93
Arizona Department of Education	65
Betty Jo Zachmeier (Mom)	iii,ix,xi,xii
Big Brothers Big Sisters	65,66,107,108,136
Bill Zachmeier (Dad)	iii,ix,xii
Billy Graham	1
Blue Öyster Cult	x,28,30,31
Bob Hope	81
Bob Miller	90
Boys & Girls Clubs of America	46,48,49,53,55,58,59,67,68,78,80,85,129
Bruce Hammer	ix,40,41,52-54,56,58,59,136
Bryan Pellican	ix
Buck Dharma	32
C. Hoppe	133
Camden Garcia	x,36,39-42,136
Camille Zachmeier	ix,xi,20,23,101,122,128
Carol Garcia	x,40
Catherine Alameda	x,31
Chace Foster	10,18
Cindi Blackwood	ix,96,98-102,136
Debbie Turner	x,31,136
Dreams Foundation, Inc	92,93,136
Dreams Realty	91
Eric Bloom	x,31,32
Franklin D. Roosevelt	43

A DAILY DIFFERENCE

Gena Foster	x,10-15,18,128,136
George Pradel	70
George Washington	67
Gil Garcia	x,40
Golden State Realty Inc	53
Harold Copenhaver	x,23
Hazel Copenhaver	x,23
Henry Ford	127
Humane Society	81
Jack London	75
Jeff Gordon	39
Joann Bersell	x,31,136
Joel Trupiano	x,128
John Fox	x,6,7,136
John P Bell Family Foundation	38
John Yacenda	92
Jules Radino	32
Julie Benson	x,31
Junior Achievement	110,111,116,117
Kathy Bell	X,116
Kathy Dirkschneider	x,23
Ken Blevins	x,47
Kim Moss	x,31
Lauren Border	x,106-110,136
Lauren Duffy	x,31
Lester Cox	ix,64,65,67,136
Linda Searfoss	66
Lizzie Bell	x,36-38,40,42,116,136
Make-A-Wish Foundation	x,28,32,33,36,39,40,44,53, 55,64,125,136
Malcolm Stevenson Forbes	61
Mike Bell	X,116
Mike Zachmeier	ix
Miley Cyrus	38
Miley Pickell	16,17

INDEX

Mission of Hope Cancer Fund	14,16
Moms with a Common Bond	100
Monta Crane	35
Montlure Camp	x,20-25
Nancy Braun	ix,78-82,136
Naomi Moon	x,30
Naperville Responds	70-72
Napoleon Hill	6
National Marrow Registry	37
National REO Brokers Association	44,64
Nevada Check Up	89,90
Nick Ryan	68,69
Norman Macewan	9
Optimist Club	128-130
Pacific Arizona Realty	64
Pat Koch	ix,84-86,87,136
Patricia Cox	64,65,67,136
PMH Financial	x,47
Ramsey Fahel	x,2,116,136
Read Across America	107
REO4Kids	Ix,44-50,52,53,55,68,78,86,93,97,136
REObroker.com	x,44
Richard Braunsteing	103
Roger Peet	ix
Ron Gamble	x,22,136
Ryan Hill Realty	70-73
Samuel Johnson	109
Sarah Carmona	92
Scott Graff	67
Scott Reed	51
Seneca	27
Showcase Realty	78
Steven Blackwood	ix,96-102,136
Stewart Title	31, 33

A DAILY DIFFERENCE

Teresa Ryan	ix,70,71,74,75,136
Terry Rasner-Yacenda	ix,90-92,136
Think and Grow Rich	6
Thomas Fuller	iii
Todd Dirkschneider	x,23
Tom Moon	x,30,44
Tori Bentley	x,31
Tortolita Presbyterian	22
United Way	123
Victor Hugo	137

ABOUT THE AUTHOR

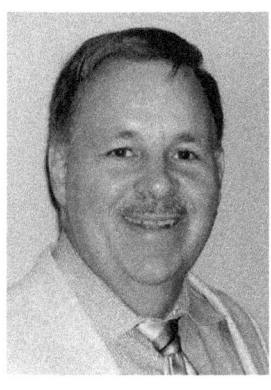

Bob Zachmeier was born and raised in Mandan, North Dakota. His parents taught by example that determination and a strong work ethic could achieve almost any goal.

As the third of six children, Zachmeier learned early in life to become self-reliant. At the age of sixteen, he owned a fireworks business, complete with billboard and radio advertising. The business helped fund his college education and that of several of his siblings.

He became a part-time real estate agent in 2000 at the age of forty. In 2002, he was earning enough from real estate investments to leave his job and end a twenty-two-year career in the defense electronics industry. In 2004, Zachmeier and his wife, Camille, founded Win3 Realty in Tucson, Arizona. The name reflects their desire to create a win-win-win situation for their clients, the agents and staff in their company, and the community. They actively support several children's charities and in 2010 received the "Spirit of Philanthropy" award from the Association of Fundraising Professionals.

In 2009, Zachmeier and other real estate brokers across the United States founded REO4Kids, a national network of top-producing real estate brokers with a "pay it forward" attitude. The group supports children's charities by holding fund raising events and donating a portion of each commission. From May, 2009, through December, 2011, REO4Kids members donated or raised more than $600,000 for children's charities. As of February, 2012, the group consists of 24 brokers in 13 states.

By sharing his experience and practical advice as a real estate broker, trainer, college instructor, author, and lecturer, Bob Zachmeier has helped thousands of people improve their financial well-being. He has written five books; *Upside Up Real Estate Investing, Sold On Change!, Answers From Experts on Buying a Home, Answers From Experts on Selling a Home, and A Daily Difference*. For information visit: **www.outoftheboxbooks.com**. You can contact the author via e-mail at: **bob@bobzachmeier.com**.

www.ingramcontent.com/pod-product-compliance
Lightning Source LLC
Chambersburg PA
CBHW032050150426
43194CB00006B/480